T0227310

Pulmonary Hypertension

Editor

RONALD J. OUDIZ

CARDIOLOGY CLINICS

www.cardiology.theclinics.com

Consulting Editors
ROSARIO FREEMAN
JORDAN M. PRUTKIN
DAVID M. SHAVELLE
AUDREY H. WU

August 2016 • Volume 34 • Number 3

ELSEVIER

1600 John F. Kennedy Boulevard • Suite 1800 • Philadelphia, Pennsylvania, 19103-2899

http://www.theclinics.com

CARDIOLOGY CLINICS Volume 34, Number 3
August 2016 ISSN 0733-8651, ISBN-13: 978-0-323-45959-4

Editor: Lauren Boyle
Developmental Editor: Alison Swety

Cardiology Clinics (ISSN 0733-8651) is published quarterly by Elsevier Inc., 360 Park Avenue South, New York, NY 10010-1710. Months of issue are February, May, August, and November. Business and Editorial Offices: 1600 John F. Kennedy Blvd., Ste. 1800, Philadelphia, PA 19103-2899. Customer Service Office: 3251 Riverport Lane, Maryland Heights, MO 63043. Periodicals post-age paid at New York, NY and additional mailing offices. Subscription prices are $320.00 per year for US individuals, $581.00 per year for US institutions, $100.00 per year for US students and residents, $390.00 per year for Canadian individuals, $729.00 per year for Canadian institutions, $455.00 per year for international individuals, $729.00 per year for international institutions and $220.00 per year for Canadian and international students/residents. To receive student/resident rate, orders must be accompanied by name of affiliated institution, data of term, and the *signature* of program/residency coordinator on institution letterhead. Orders will be billed at individual rate until proof of status is received. Foreign air speed delivery is included in all *Clinics* subscription prices. All prices are subject to change without notice. **POSTMASTER:** Send address changes to *Cardiology Clinics*, Elsevier Health Sciences Division, Subscription Customer Service, 3251 Riverport Lane, Maryland Heights, MO 63043. **Customer Service: 1-800-654-2452 (U.S. and Canada); 314-447-8871 (outside U.S. and Canada). Fax: 314-447-8029. E-mail: journalscustomerservice-usa@ elsevier.com (for print support); journalsonlinesupport-usa@elsevier.com (for online support).**

Reprints. For copies of 100 or more, of articles in this publication, please contact the Commercial Reprints Department, Elsevier Inc., 360 Park Avenue South, New York, NY 10010-1710. Tel.: 212-633-3874; Fax: 212-633-3820; E-mail: reprints@elsevier.com.

Cardiology Clinics is also published in Spanish by McGraw-Hill Interamericana Editores S. A., P.O. Box 5-237, 06500, Mexico D. F., Mexico; in Portuguese by Reichmann and Alfonso Editores Rio de Janeiro, Brazil; and in Greek by Dimitrios P. Lagos, 8 Pondon Street, GR115-28 Ilissia, Greece.

Cardiology Clinics is covered in *MEDLINE/PubMed (Index Medicus), Excerpta Medica, The Cumulative Index to Nursing and Allied Health Literature* (CINAHL).

Contributors

EDITORIAL BOARD

ROSARIO FREEMAN, MD, MS, FACC
Associate Professor of Medicine; Director,
Coronary Care Unit; Director,
Echocardiography Laboratory, University of
Washington Medical Center, Seattle,
Washington

JORDAN M. PRUTKIN, MD, MHS, FHRS
Assistant Professor of Medicine, Division of
Cardiology/Electrophysiology, University of
Washington Medical Center, Seattle,
Washington

DAVID M. SHAVELLE, MD, FACC, FSCAI
Associate Professor, Keck School of Medicine;
Director, General Cardiovascular Fellowship
Program; Director, Cardiac Catheterization
Laboratory, Los Angeles County + USC
Medical Center; Division of Cardiovascular
Medicine, University of Southern California,
Los Angeles, California

AUDREY H. WU, MD
Assistant Professor, Internal Medicine,
University of Michigan, Ann Arbor, Michigan

EDITOR

RONALD J. OUDIZ, MD, FACP, FACC, FCCP
Professor of Medicine, The David Geffen
School of Medicine at UCLA; Director,
Liu Center for Pulmonary Hypertension,
Division of Cardiology, Department of
Medicine, Los Angeles Biomedical Research
Institute at Harbor–UCLA Medical Center,
Torrance, California

AUTHORS

JAMIL A. ABOULHOSN, MD, FACC, FSCAI
Director, Ahmanson/UCLA Adult Congenital
Heart Disease Center, Streisand/American
Heart Association Endowed Chair; Associate
Professor of Medicine and Pediatrics, David
Geffen School of Medicine at UCLA,
Los Angeles, California

PAULINO ALVAREZ, MD
Department of Cardiology, Methodist DeBakey
Heart and Vascular Center, Houston Methodist
Hospital, Houston, Texas

CHRISTOPHER F. BARNETT, MD, MPH
Director, Pulmonary Hypertension Program,
Medstar Heart and Vascular Institute,
Washington, DC; Critical Care Medicine

Department, National Institutes of Health,
Bethesda, Maryland

MURALI M. CHAKINALA, MD
Director, WUSM – BJH Pulmonary
Hypertension Care Center; Associate
Professor of Medicine, Division of Pulmonary
and Critical Care Medicine, Washington
University School of Medicine, St Louis,
Missouri

CRAIG B. CLARK, DO, FHFSA
Associate Professor of Medicine, Division of
Cardiology, Department of Internal Medicine,
Des Moines University, Iowa Heart Center,
Des Moines, Iowa

TERESA DE MARCO, MD
Director of Advanced Heart Failure and
Pulmonary Hypertension and Medical
Director of Heart Transplantation; Professor,
Division of Cardiology, Department of
Medicine, University of California San
Francisco, San Francisco, California

MARIBETH DUNCAN, APRN
Program Coordinator, WUSM – BJH
Pulmonary Hypertension Care Center,
Barnes-Jewish Hospital, St Louis, Missouri

MARDI GOMBERG-MAITLAND, MD, MSc
Section of Cardiology, Department of
Medicine, University of Chicago Medical
Center; Associate Professor of Medicine,
Pulmonary Hypertension Program,
Cardiovascular Division, University of Chicago
Medical Center, Chicago, Illinois

EVELYN M. HORN, MD
Professor of Clinical Medicine; Director of
Advanced Heart Failure, Mechanical
Circulatory Assist and Pulmonary Hypertension
Programs, Division of Cardiology, Perkin Heart
Failure Center, Weill Cornell Medical Center,
New York, New York

DUNBAR IVY, MD
Professor of Pediatrics; Chief and Selby's
Chair of Pediatric Cardiology, Section of
Pediatric Cardiology, Children's Hospital
Colorado, University of Colorado School of
Medicine, Aurora, Colorado

MUNIR JANMOHAMMED, MD
Advanced Heart Failure and Pulmonary
Hypertension Program; Assistant Professor,
Division of Cardiology, Department of
Medicine, University of California San
Francisco, San Francisco, California

SARA KALANTARI, MD
Section of Cardiology, Department of
Medicine, University of Chicago Medical
Center, Chicago, Illinois

NICK H. KIM, MD
Clinical Professor of Medicine; Director of
Pulmonary Vascular Medicine, Division of
Pulmonary and Critical Care Medicine,
University of California, San Diego, La Jolla,
California

JAMES R. KLINGER, MD
Professor of Medicine, Division of Pulmonary,
Sleep and Critical Care Medicine, Alpert
Medical School of Brown University, Rhode
Island Hospital, Ambulatory Patient Center,
Providence, Rhode Island

RONALD J. OUDIZ, MD, FACP, FACC, FCCP
Professor of Medicine, The David Geffen
School of Medicine at UCLA; Director,
Liu Center for Pulmonary Hypertension,
Division of Cardiology, Department of
Medicine, Los Angeles Biomedical Research
Institute at Harbor–UCLA Medical Center,
Torrance, California

MYUNG H. PARK, MD
Chief, Division of Heart Failure and Transplant,
Department of Cardiology, Methodist DeBakey
Heart and Vascular Center, Houston Methodist
Hospital, Houston, Texas

KURT W. PRINS, MD, PhD
Cardiovascular Division, University of
Minnesota Medical School, Minneapolis,
Minnesota

TODD S. ROTH, MD
Co-Director Memorial Cardiac and Vascular
Institute, Joe DiMaggio Children's Hospital,
Adult Congenital Heart Disease Center,
Hollywood, Florida

JANA SVETLICHNAYA, MD, MSc
Advanced Heart Failure and Pulmonary
Hypertension Program; Fellow, Division of
Cardiology, Department of Medicine,
University of California San Francisco,
San Francisco, California

THENAPPAN THENAPPAN, MD
Assistant Professor of Medicine, Section of
Advanced Heart Failure and Pulmonary
Hypertension, Cardiovascular Division,
University of Minnesota Medical School,
Minneapolis, Minnesota

JOEL WIRTH, MD
Associate Clinical Professor of Medicine,
Department of Medicine, Tufts University
School of Medicine, Boston, Massachusetts;
Director, Division of Pulmonary and Critical
Care Medicine, Maine Medical Center,
Portland, Maine

Contents

> The classification of pulmonary hypertension (PH) is an attempt to define subtypes of PH based on clinical presentation, underlying physiology, and treatment implications. Five groups of PH have been defined, and the classification scheme has been refined over the years to guide clinicians in the diagnosis and management of PH. Understanding the classification of PH is paramount before embarking on a work-up of patients with PH or suspected PH because treatment and outcome can vary greatly.

> Pulmonary arterial hypertension (PAH) is a debilitating disease characterized by pathologic remodeling of the resistance pulmonary arteries, ultimately leading to right ventricular (RV) failure and death. In this article we discuss the definition of PAH, the initial epidemiology based on the National Institutes of Health Registry, and the updated epidemiology gleaned from contemporary registries, pathogenesis of pulmonary vascular dysfunction and proliferation, and RV failure in PAH.

 Video content accompanies this article at http://www.cardiology.theclinics.com.

> Pulmonary arterial hypertension (PAH) is a specific, rare disease characterized by a well-described pattern of pulmonary vascular remodeling. The elevated pulmonary artery pressure in PAH results in increased right ventricular afterload, which, if untreated, leads rapidly to right ventricular failure and death. Recent marked expansion in knowledge about PAH has resulted in the development of effective therapies that improve quality of life and survival. However, delays in diagnosis and suboptimal treatment remain significant barriers to achieving optimal patient outcomes. Continued success in raising PAH awareness, earlier diagnosis, and the availability of new therapies mean a promising future for PAH patients.

> Pulmonary arterial hypertension in congenital heart disease (PAH-CHD) is a frequent complication in adults with congenital heart disease. Regardless of etiology, the optimal treatment strategy for this difficult population is challenging. The new frontier of targeted PAH therapies has demonstrated improved functional capacity in the

various phenotypes of PAH-CHD, with work currently in progress scrutinizing outcomes. In those who fail conventional medical therapy, heart and heart-lung (block) transplantation become the final therapeutic options, with the role of ventricular assist devices and the total artificial heart still under investigation in this group.

Pulmonary hypertension from left heart disease (PH-LHD) is the most common form of PH, defined as mean pulmonary artery pressure $\geq$25 mm Hg and pulmonary artery wedge pressure $\geq$15 mm Hg. PH-LHD development is associated with more severe left-sided disease and its presence portends a poor prognosis, particularly once right ventricular failure develops. Treatment remains focused on the underlying LHD and despite initial enthusiasm for PH-specific therapies, most studies have been disappointing and their routine clinical use cannot be recommended. More work is urgently needed to better understand the pathophysiology underlying this disease and to develop effective therapeutic strategies.

Pulmonary hypertension (PH) associated with chronic lung disease (WHO group 3) is the second leading cause of PH and is associated with increased morbidity and mortality. Elevation of pulmonary arterial pressure (PAP) is usually moderate and correlates with severity of lung disease. In a small minority, PAP may approach that seen in WHO group 1 pulmonary arterial hypertension (PAH). Current medications for treating PAH have not shown benefit in controlled trials of group 3 PH and their routine use is discouraged. Patients with severe group 3 PH should be considered for referral to expert centers or entry into clinical trials.

Chronic thromboembolic pulmonary hypertension (CTEPH) is a serious but treatable complication of pulmonary embolism. Proper diagnosis and referral are critical, as pulmonary thromboendarterectomy offers the possibility of a cure. For patients with CTEPH deemed inoperable, new and effective treatments have emerged to help fill this unmet need.

Pulmonary hypertension is a complex disorder with multiple etiologies; the World Health Organization classification system divides pulmonary hypertension patients into 5 groups based on the underlying cause and mechanism. Group 5 pulmonary hypertension is a heterogeneous group of diseases that encompasses pulmonary hypertension secondary to multifactorial mechanisms. For many of the diseases, the true incidence, etiology, and treatment remain uncertain. This article reviews the epidemiology, pathogenesis, and management of many of the group 5 pulmonary hypertension disease states.

Pulmonary Hypertension in Children 451

Dunbar Ivy

The prevalence of PH is increasing in the pediatric population, because of improved recognition and increased survival of patients, and remains a significant cause of morbidity and mortality. Recent studies have improved the understanding of pediatric PH, but management remains challenging because of a lack of evidence-based clinical trials. The growing contribution of developmental lung disease requires dedicated research to explore the use of existing therapies as well as the creation of novel therapies. Adequate study of pediatric PH will require multicenter collaboration due to the small numbers of patients, multifactorial disease causes, and practice variability.

Special Situations in Pulmonary Hypertension: Pregnancy and Right Ventricular Failure 473

Jana Svetlichnaya, Munir Janmohammed, and Teresa De Marco

Despite rapid advances in medical therapy, pregnancy and right ventricular (RV) failure predicts a poor prognosis in patients with pulmonary arterial hypertension. Evidence-based therapy for pulmonary arterial hypertension should be initiated early in the disease course to decrease RV wall stress and prevent RV remodeling and fibrosis. In patients with acutely decompensated RV failure, an aggressive and multifaceted approach must be used; a thorough search for triggering factors for the decompensation is a key part of the successful management strategy. Patients with refractory RV failure who are not candidates for surgical intervention should be referred to palliative care to maximize quality of life and symptom relief.

Managing the Patient with Pulmonary Hypertension: Specialty Care Centers, Coordinated Care, and Patient Support 489

Murali M. Chakinala, Maribeth Duncan, and Joel Wirth

Pulmonary hypertension remains a challenging condition to diagnose and manage. Decentralized care for pulmonary arterial hypertension (PAH) has led to shortcomings in the diagnosis and management of PAH. The Pulmonary Hypertension Association–sponsored Pulmonary Hypertension Care Center program is designed to recognize specialty centers capable of providing multidisciplinary and comprehensive care of PAH. Ideally, Pulmonary Hypertension Care Centers will comanage PAH patients with community-based practitioners and address the growing needs of this emerging population of long-term PAH patients.

CARDIOLOGY CLINICS

ISSUE OF RELATED INTEREST

Cardiac Electrophysiology Clinics, March 2016 (Vol. 8, No. 1)
Interpretation of Complex Arrhythmias: A Case-Based Approach
Melvin Scheinman, *Editor*
Available at: http://www.cardiacep.theclinics.com/

THE CLINICS ARE AVAILABLE ONLINE!
Access your subscription at:
www.theclinics.com

Preface
Pulmonary Hypertension

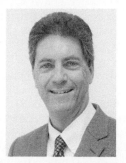

Ronald J. Oudiz, MD, FACP, FACC, FCCP
Editor

It is an exciting time for scientists and clinicians in the field of pulmonary hypertension (PH) and right-sided heart failure today. The discipline has developed and matured into one that has seen more than a dozen drugs approved to treat pulmonary arterial hypertension (PAH) over the past several years. In addition, PH awareness programs have flourished, and the field is poised to see the development of new treatment targets that may further improve outcomes in PAH, and possibly (finally) will do so in other forms of PH.

This issue of *Cardiology Clinics* thoroughly covers the science, clinical findings, and diagnostic and treatment approaches of each of the 5 subgroups of PH as we know and define them today. Special situations unique to PH patients are addressed as well. The experts chosen to author each article were selected based on their experience and their contributions to the field. We hope that readers of this comprehensive work will benefit from their expertise and that they will better understand the nuances and peculiarities of PH, an often poorly understood and frustrating disorder.

Ronald J. Oudiz, MD, FACP, FACC, FCCP
The David Geffen School of Medicine at UCLA
Liu Center for Pulmonary Hypertension
Division of Cardiology, Department of Medicine
Los Angeles Biomedical Research Institute
at Harbor–UCLA Medical Center
1124 West Carson Street
Torrance, CA 90502, USA

E-mail address:
roudiz@labiomed.org

Cardiol Clin 34 (2016) ix
http://dx.doi.org/10.1016/j.ccl.2016.05.001
0733-8651/16/$ – see front matter © 2016 Published by Elsevier Inc.

Classification of Pulmonary Hypertension

Ronald J. Oudiz, MD

KEYWORDS

• Pulmonary hypertension • Classification • WHO Group

KEY POINTS

• Pulmonary hypertension comes in many forms.
• The classification scheme used to classify pulmonary hypertension is in part based on clinical presentation, in part based on physiology, and in part based on treatment implications.
• Treatment can vary greatly depending on the type of pulmonary hypertension, thus proper diagnosis and classification are key.

The classification of pulmonary hypertension (PH) was first published in contemporary works dating back to the 1950s.[1] More recently, expert consensus proceedings have attempted to better define and refine a classification scheme that is in part based on clinical presentation, in part based on physiology, and in part based on treatment implications.[2]

Box 1[2] shows the latest clinical classification of PH put forth by the proceedings of the most recent world meeting on PH that took place in Nice, France, in 2013. This classification, updated from the world meetings in Dana Point, California, in 2008, made some minor changes to the prior classification to allow for newer discoveries since 2008, and to accommodate a consensus rethinking of the various subtypes.

As discussed later, the various types of PH can differ greatly in their underlying pathophysiology, and particularly in their treatment implications. However, their clinical presentations, at least initially, can be very similar. Dyspnea, fatigue, and syncope are all common symptoms of patients presenting with PH because impaired pulmonary blood flow during exercise impairs systemic blood flow,[3] and also because the right ventricle bears the brunt of the insult[4]; this is regardless of the origin of the PH.

Group I PH is rare form of precapillary PH known as pulmonary arterial hypertension (PAH), with an incidence of less than 10 per million per year by some reports (see Prins KW, Thenappan T: WHO Group I Pulmonary Hypertension: Epidemiology and Pathophysiology, in this issue; and Barnet CF, Alvarez P, Park MH: Pulmonary Arterial Hypertension: Diagnosis and Treatment, in this issue).[5] It is a diagnosis in which known causes of PH are excluded, and represents a poorly understood consequence of an intrinsic abnormality of the pulmonary circulation that leads to an increase in pulmonary vascular resistance, right heart failure, and untimely death.

In its purest form, PAH with no associated condition is known as idiopathic PAH. However, several conditions, such as connective tissue disease, human immunodeficiency virus infection, and portal hypertension, seem to predispose patients to developing PAH more commonly, although still rarely. In addition, several genes have been identified in a heritable form of PH that phenotypically mimics idiopathic PAH.

In recent years, several treatments have been developed to treat group I PH. It is important to understand that many of these drugs have been studied in other forms of PH; that is, group II and group III PH (discussed further later). In these studies, the treatments were found to either be neutral or negative, with a poor risk/benefit ratio. Therefore, it is extremely important to be as certain as possible that the correct assignment of PH

Division of Cardiology, Department of Medicine, Los Angeles Biomedical Research Institute, Harbor-UCLA Medical Center, Torrance, CA 90502, USA
E-mail address: roudiz@labiomed.org

Cardiol Clin 34 (2016) 359–361
http://dx.doi.org/10.1016/j.ccl.2016.04.009
0733-8651/16/$ – see front matter © 2016 Elsevier Inc. All rights reserved.

cardiology.theclinics.com

Box 1
Updated classification of PH

1. Pulmonary arterial hypertension

   a. Idiopathic PAH

   b. Heritable PAH

      i. BMPR2

      ii. ALK-1, ENG, SMAD9, CAV1, KCNK3

      iii. Unknown

   c. Drug and toxin induced

   d. Associated with:

      i. Connective tissue disease

      ii. HIV infection

      iii. Portal hypertension

      iv. Congenital heart diseases

      v. Schistosomiasis

1'. Pulmonary veno-occlusive disease and/or pulmonary capillary hemangiomatosis

1". Persistent PH of the newborn

2. PH caused by left heart disease

   a. Left ventricular systolic dysfunction

   b. Left ventricular diastolic dysfunction

   c. Valvular disease

   d. Congenital/acquired left heart inflow/outflow tract obstruction and congenital cardiomyopathies

3. Pulmonary hypertension caused by lung diseases and/or hypoxia

   a. Chronic obstructive pulmonary disease

   b. Interstitial lung disease

   c. Other pulmonary diseases with mixed restrictive and obstructive pattern

   d. Sleep-disordered breathing

   e. Alveolar hypoventilation disorders

   f. Chronic exposure to high altitude

   g. Developmental lung diseases

4. Chronic thromboembolic pulmonary hypertension

5. PH with unclear multifactorial mechanisms

   a. Hematologic disorders: chronic hemolytic anemia, myeloproliferative disorders, splenectomy

   b. Systemic disorders: sarcoidosis, pulmonary histiocytosis, lymphangioleiomyomatosis

   c. Metabolic disorders: glycogen storage disease, Gaucher disease, thyroid disorders

   d. Others: tumoral obstruction, fibrosing mediastinitis, chronic renal failure, segmental PH

The Fifth World Symposium on Pulmonary Hypertension, Nice 2013. Main modifications to the previous Dana Point classification are in bold.
Abbreviations: BMPR, bone morphogenetic protein receptor type II; CAV1, caveolin-1; ENG, endoglin; HIV, human immunodeficiency virus; PAH, pulmonary arterial hypertension.
From Simonneau G, Gatzoulis MA, Adatia I, et al. Updated clinical classification of pulmonary hypertension. J Am Coll Cardiol 2013;62(25 Suppl):D36; with permission.

classification is given, especially when attempting to classify a patient with PH to group I.

In general, when cardiologists in the Western world encounter patients with PH, most commonly they are seeing PH related to impaired blood flow distal to the precapillary circulation; that is, to the systemic side of the circulatory system. This condition is often referred to as pulmonary venous hypertension (PVH) and is classified as group II PH (see Clark CB, Horn EM: Group II PH: Pulmonary Venous Hypertension: Epidemiology and Pathophysiology, in this issue). In group II PH, PVH may be caused by left-sided myocardial disease or left-sided cardiac valve disease, and it is treated entirely differently from other groups of PH. Namely, the underlying cause of the PVH is treated with therapies to address the physiologic derangements that accompany left-side heart disease; that is, fixing the valve disease, supporting myocardial dysfunction with afterload reduction and beta blockers, and so forth. None of the therapies currently used for ameliorating PVH in patients with pulmonary I hypertension have been shown to be beneficial.

Pulmonologists in the Western world typically see PH related to hypoxic lung disease, classified as group III PH (see Klinger JR: Group III PH Pulmonary Hypertension Associated with Lung Disease: Epidemiology, Pathophysiology, and Treatments, in this issue). These patients generally have identifiable factors responsible for their underlying hypoxia. Although their hemodynamic abnormalities share similarities with group I PH (high pulmonary vascular resistance with normal pulmonary capillary wedge pressure), it is the hypoxia that drives the PH in patients with group III PH. This condition is in contrast with the idiopathic nature of the intrinsic precapillary circulatory abnormalities seen in group I PH. In group III PH, treatments are designed to improve the underlying airways disease using supportive therapies such as long-term oxygen therapy and rehabilitative exercise to help patients compensate for their impairment in exercise tolerance, and targeted medical therapy where applicable.

Group IV PH, chronic thromboembolic PH (CTEPH), is a disease specific to patients who develop increased pulmonary vascular resistance caused by the development of chronic pulmonary emboli. As with patients with group I PH, it is important to recognize the presence of chronic thromboembolic disease in symptomatic patients because the disease is treatable (see Kim NH: Group IV PH: CTEPH: Epidemiology, Pathophysiology, and Treatment, in this issue). Failure to recognize the presence of CTEPH could lead to errors in diagnosis, and missed opportunities for treatment and possibly complete reversal of the PH.

In addition, group V PH represents a frustrating if not controversial mixture of PH types that do not fit nicely into groups I to IV (see Tannenbaum SK, Gomberg-Maitland M: Group 5 Pulmonary Hypertension: the Orphan's Orphan Disease, in this issue). In many cases, group 5 PH might be related to multifactorial mechanisms, such as those producing disease of the pulmonary circulation directly, combined with those that passively increase pulmonary arterial pressure. Still other cases include those with localized or systemic diseases that themselves are poorly understood. These patients cannot reliably be compartmentalized into any of the other PH groups and represent an area for ongoing study, both in the pathophysiologic nature of their PH-causing mechanisms and in the search for treatments that could ameliorate symptoms and/or improve outcomes in this subset.

Throughout the articles in this series, it is important to understand the basics of the PH classification scheme put forth by consensus. It is particularly important to keep in mind that, although group I PH is the rarest of all types of PH, if the disease is missed and left untreated, the outcome can be extremely grave.

REFERENCES

1. Edwards JE. Classification of chronic pulmonary hypertension. Med Clin North Am 1958;42:1037–45.
2. Simonneau G, Gatzoulis MA, Adatia I, et al. Updated clinical classification of pulmonary hypertension. J Am Coll Cardiol 2013;62:D34–41.
3. Sun XG, Hansen JE, Oudiz RJ, et al. Exercise pathophysiology in patients with primary pulmonary hypertension. Circulation 2001;104:429–35.
4. Vonk-Noordegraaf A, Haddad F, Chin KM, et al. Right heart adaptation to pulmonary arterial hypertension: physiology and pathobiology. J Am Coll Cardiol 2013;62:D22–33.
5. Humbert M, Sitbon O, Chaouat A, et al. Pulmonary arterial hypertension in France: results from a national registry. Am J Respir Crit Care Med 2006; 173:1023–30.

World Health Organization Group I Pulmonary Hypertension
Epidemiology and Pathophysiology

Kurt W. Prins, MD, PhD[a], Thenappan Thenappan, MD[b],*

KEYWORDS

- Pulmonary arterial hypertension • Epidemiology • Right ventricle • Pulmonary vasculature
- Pathophysiology

KEY POINTS

- Pulmonary arterial hypertension (PAH) is characterized by pathologic vascular remodeling resulting in elevated pulmonary artery pressures and eventual right ventricular (RV) dysfunction.
- PAH remains a rare disease with a female predominance and an evolving epidemiology as our awareness of the disease improves.
- The pathologic changes in the pulmonary vasculature include pulmonary vascular dysfunction and excessive proliferation, with multiple molecular mechanisms contributing to both phenotypes.
- RV is the major predictor of outcomes in PAH, but our knowledge about RV failure in PAH is limited.
- Available evidence on RV dysfunction suggests several pathways converge to promote RV failure in PAH.

DEFINITION AND CLASSIFICATION

Pulmonary hypertension (PH) is defined as mean pulmonary arterial pressure (PAP) measured by right heart catheterization of 25 mm Hg or higher at rest.[1] The most recent World Health Organization (WHO) classification has categorized PH into 5 different groups based on the underlying mechanism (**Box 1**). Pulmonary arterial hypertension (PAH) represents group I within the WHO classification. The following is the hemodynamic-based definition of PAH:

- Mean PAP ≥25 mm Hg
- Pulmonary capillary wedge pressure (PCWP) <15 mm Hg
- Pulmonary vascular resistance (PVR) ≥3 Wood units.

PAH includes a group of disorders with similar pulmonary vascular pathophysiological mechanisms and clinical characteristics. PAH can be idiopathic (IPAH), hereditable (HPAH), or associated with other conditions, such as connective tissue disease, congenital heart disease, portal hypertension, human immunodeficiency virus (HIV) infection, anorexigen exposure, or schistosomiasis.

EPIDEMIOLOGY
The National Institutes of Health Registry

The landmark National Institutes of Health (NIH) registry was a multicenter registry that collected

Disclosures: None.

Funding: T. Thenappan was funded by AHA Scientist Development Grant 15SDG25560048 and K.W. Prins was funded by National Institutes of Health F32 grant HL129554.

[a] Cardiovascular Division, University of Minnesota Medical School, 420 Delaware Street Southeast, Minneapolis, MN 55455, USA; [b] Section of Advanced Heart Failure and Pulmonary Hypertension, Cardiovascular Division, University of Minnesota Medical School, 420 Delaware Street Southeast, Minneapolis, MN 55455, USA

* Corresponding author.

E-mail address: tthenapp@umn.edu

Cardiol Clin 34 (2016) 363–374

http://dx.doi.org/10.1016/j.ccl.2016.04.001

Box 1
World Health Organization classification of pulmonary hypertension subtypes

1. Pulmonary arterial hypertension (PAH)
   a. Idiopathic PAH
   b. Heritable PAH
      i. BMPR2
      ii. ALK-1, ENG, *SMAD9, CAV1, KCNK3*
      iii. Unknown
   c. Drug and toxin induced
   d. Associated with
      i. Connective tissue disease
      ii. Human immunodeficiency virus infection
      iii. Portal hypertension
      iv. Congenital heart diseases
      v. Schistosomiasis
1′ Pulmonary veno-occlusive disease and/or pulmonary capillary
   Hemangiomatosis
1″ Persistent pulmonary hypertension of the newborn (PPHN)
2. Pulmonary hypertension due to left heart disease
   a. Left ventricular systolic dysfunction
   b. Left ventricular diastolic dysfunction
   c. Valvular disease
   d. *Congenital/acquired left heart inflow/outflow tract obstruction and congenital cardiomyopathies*
3. Pulmonary hypertension due to lung diseases and/or hypoxia
   a. Chronic obstructive pulmonary disease
   b. Interstitial lung disease
   c. Other pulmonary diseases with mixed restrictive and obstructive pattern
   d. Sleep-disordered breathing
   e. Alveolar hypoventilation disorders
   f. Chronic exposure to high altitude
   g. *Developmental lung diseases*
4. Chronic thromboembolic pulmonary hypertension (CTEPH)
5. Pulmonary hypertension with unclear multifactorial mechanisms
   a. *Hematologic disorders: chronic hemolytic anemia*, myeloproliferative disorders, splenectomy
   b. *Systemic disorders: sarcoidosis, pulmonary histiocytosis, Lymphangioleiomyomatosis*
   c. Metabolic disorders: glycogen storage disease, Gaucher disease, thyroid disorders
   d. Others: tumoral obstruction, fibrosing mediastinitis, chronic renal failure, segmental pulmonary hypertension

data prospectively from 1981 to 1985 from 32 centers in the United States.[2] A total of 187 patients with idiopathic, hereditary, or anorexigen-associated PAH were included. PAH was defined as mean PAP of 25 mm Hg or higher at rest or 30 mm Hg or higher with exercise and PCWP lower than 12 mm Hg. The mean age at presentation was 36 ± 15 years and the most patients were women. The distribution of patients based on race was 85.4% white, 12.3% African American, and 2.3%

Hispanic. The mean time interval between onset of symptoms and diagnosis was 2 years. Dyspnea was the most common presenting symptom followed by fatigue and syncope. Patients in the registry had severe PAH based on hemodynamics with a mean PAP of 60 ± 18 mm Hg, a PVR index of 26 ± 14 Wood Units, and a cardiac index (CI) of 2.3 ± 0.9 L/min/m². Treatment consisted of diuretics, digoxin, and supplemental nasal oxygen and, in a minority of cases, anticoagulation with warfarin. PAH-specific vasodilator therapy was not available, but a small number of patients were treated with calcium-channel blockers and/or hydralazine. The estimated median survival was 2.8 years with a 1-year survival of 68%, 3-year survival of 48%, and a 5-year survival of 34%.[3] The registry developed a regression equation to predict survival based on the baseline hemodynamics (mean right atrial pressure, CI, and mean PAP) at the time of diagnosis, and it was subsequently used in many therapeutic trials to demonstrate improved survival in patients with idiopathic or hereditary PAH by comparing the observed versus the survival rates predicted by the equation. However, the NIH equation underestimates survival in the current era and is therefore no longer valid.[4]

Contemporary Pulmonary Arterial Hypertension Registries

Since the NIH registry, there has been a remarkable progress in both the understanding of the pathophysiology and treatment options of PAH. Unlike the NIH registry, the current WHO classification of PAH includes IPAH, HPH, anorexigen-associated PH, PH associated with connective tissue disease, congenital heart disease, portal hypertension, and HIV infection. Furthermore, the Food and Drug Administration has approved 12 drugs for the treatment of PAH over the past 2 decades.[5] Due to these changes, several contemporary registries were developed to update both the epidemiologic and prognostic data of PAH. There are several differences between these registries, including the time period of enrollment, etiology of PAH patient population enrolled (idiopathic/heritable PAH vs associated PAH), study design (retrospective vs prospective), and study cohort (incident cases vs prevalent cases). **Table 1** describes the 11 major PAH registries.[2,6–15]

Epidemiology of Pulmonary Arterial Hypertension in the Modern Era

Although the incidence and prevalence of PAH in North America are unknown, studies from Scotland and France revealed an incidence of 2.5 to 7.1 cases per million and a prevalence ranging from 5 to 52 per million adults.[6,13] In the major PAH registries, approximately half of the patients had IPAH or HPAH and the remaining had associated PAH. Of the patients with associated PAH, the most common etiology was connective tissue disease followed by congenital heart disease.[6–8] Scleroderma was the most common connective tissue disease associated with PAH. In the French registry, there was a higher prevalence of PAH associated with anorexigen use (9.5% vs 3.0%–5.3%) and HIV infection (6.2% vs 1.0%–2.3%) compared with US-based registries.[16] In China, PAH associated with congenital heart disease was the predominant cause of WHO Group I PAH, a finding that differed from all other countries.[12]

Analysis of contemporary PAH registries suggest that PAH epidemiology has changed significantly over the past 3 decades.[16] The mean age of the patients with IPAH or HPAH in the contemporary registries from the Western world ranged from 45 to 65 years, which is much higher than the NIH registry. The reason for the dramatic increase in mean age at the time of presentation is unclear, but there are several probable explanations. First, most of the modern registries enrolled predominantly prevalent cases (~85%) of PAH, which was not used in the NIH registry, which may have introduced survivor bias. However, in the incident cases in both the French registry and the PH registry of the United Kingdom and Ireland, which studied only treatment-naïve incident IPAH, HPAH, and anorexigen-associated PAH, the median age at the time of enrollment was 50 years (vs 36 years in the NIH registry) with 13.5% of the total UK and Ireland cohort older than 70 years at the time of diagnosis.[6,9] Second, there is increased awareness of PAH in the Western world due to the availability of Doppler echocardiography as a PH screening tool and the availability of effective PAH-specific therapies. Interestingly, patients in the Chinese IPAH cohort had a profile as the NIH cohort, arguing that the increased age in the Western cohort was caused by detection of PAH in older patients and not an actual change in the biological phenotype of PAH.[14] Moreover, it is also possible that the increasing age at the time of presentation was due to misclassification of PH, especially PH associated with heart failure with preserved ejection fraction (HFpEF) being misclassified as PAH due to overreliance on a single measurement of a resting PCWP.[17] These 2 clinical entities have common clinical characteristics,[18] and the differentiation between these 2 rests exclusively on PCWP value, which can be erroneous in many

Table 1
Characterization of 11 major PAH registries

Registry	Study Cohort	Number	Time Period	Study Design	Study Cohort	IPAH/HPAH vs APAH
NIH	IPAH	187	1981–1985	Prospective	Incident cases	NA
Chinese	IPAH/HPAH	72	1999–2004	Prospective	Incident cases	NA
COMPERA[a]	IPAH/HPAH	587	2007–2011	Prospective	Incident cases	NA
French	Group I PAH	674	2002–2003	Prospective	Incident and prevalent cases	39% vs 61%
Mayo	Group I PAH	484	1995–2004	Prospective	Incident and prevalent cases	—
New Chinese	Group I PAH	956	2008–2011	Prospective	Incident cases	35% vs 65%
PHC	Group I PAH	578	1982–2006	Retrospective & Prospective	Incident and prevalent cases	48% vs 52%
REVEAL	Group I PAH	3515	2006–2009	Prospective	Incident and prevalent cases	46% vs 54%
Scottish-SMR	Group I PAH	374	1986–2001	Retrospective	Incident cases	47% vs 54%
Spanish	Group I PAH CTEPH	866/162	1998–2008	Retrospective & Prospective	Incident and prevalent cases	36% vs 64%
United Kingdom and Ireland	IPAH, HPAH, and Anorexigen-APAH	482	2001–2009	—	Incident cases	98.3% vs 1.7%

Abbreviations: APAH, associated PAH; COMPERA, Comparative, Prospective Registry of Newly Initiated Therapies for Pulmonary Hypertension; CTEPH, chronic thromboembolic pulmonary hypertension; HPAH, heritable PAH; IPAH, idiopathic PAH; NIH, National Institutes of Health; PAH, pulmonary arterial hypertension; PHC, Pulmonary Hypertension Connections; REVEAL, Registry to Evaluate Early and Long-Term PAH Disease Management; SMR, Scottish Morbidity Record.
[a] COMPERA registry enrolled patients with any World Health Organization group PH. The data presented here are for the incident IPAH cohort only.

situations.[19,20] This concept is further supported by the enrollment pattern observed in the most recently completed PAH clinical trial. The Ambrisentan and Tadalafil in Patients with Pulmonary Arterial Hypertension (AMBITION) trial was a randomized, double-blind, placebo-controlled, clinical trial designed to compare the benefits of initial double combination therapy with ambrisentan and tadalafil versus monotherapy with either ambrisentan or tadalafil. The steering committee had to stop enrollment briefly and modify inclusion criteria, as the phenotype of the first 100 patients entered into this clinical trial was very similar to PH associated with HFpEF as opposed to PAH.[21]

PAH shows a female predominance with a female/male ratio of 1.7:1.0 in the NIH registry.[2] Contemporary registries of PAH also showed a female-dominant distribution, although, the female/male ratio was significantly higher in the modern US-based registries: Pulmonary Hypertension Connection (PHC) registry, 3.0:1.0; Registry to Evaluate Early and Long-Term PAH Disease Management (REVEAL) registry, 4.8:1.0; and the Mayo registry, 3.2:1.0.[16,22] The reason for the increasing female predominance, particularly in the modern US-based PAH registries, compared with the European registries, is unclear. One possible explanation is the increased use of hormone replacement therapy in the United States in the 1980s and the 1990s; however, this is a speculation and has not been tested.

Racial distribution of PAH was explored in the REVEAL registry; the patient distribution was 72.8% white, 12.2% African American, 8.9% Hispanic, 3.3% Asian or Pacific Islander, and 2.8% other or unknown. The proportion of whites in the REVEAL registry was similar to the age and sex-adjusted expected distribution of whites in the US population; however, there was overrepresentation of African American individuals (12.2% vs 10.9%) and underrepresentation of Hispanic (8.9% vs 11.5%) and Asian/Pacific Islander individuals (3.3% vs 4.3%).[16] Other contemporary US and non-US based registries lacked data on race.

Despite increasing awareness of PAH, a significant lag between the onset of symptoms and the diagnosis of PAH still exists. The mean interval between onset of symptoms and diagnosis of PAH in the contemporary registries ranged from 18 to 32 months (vs 2 years in the NIH registry).[9,23] In the REVEAL registry, 20% of patients had symptoms for more than 2 years before diagnosis. Similar to the NIH registry, most of the PAH in contemporary registries had advanced WHO functional III and IV symptoms at the time of diagnosis (56%–91%). The mean 6-minute walk distance at the time of presentation in the contemporary registries ranged from 292 ± 129 m to 382 ± 117 m. Assessment of invasive hemodynamics in patients with PAH in the contemporary registries revealed significantly elevated mean PAP and PVR with moderately reduced CI at the time of presentation, very similar to the NIH registry. Only a minority of patients (4.5%–10.0%) had a positive acute vasodilator response, and IPAH was the predominant etiology of those with a positive response. In contrast to the NIH registry, contemporary registry patients have multiple comorbidities, such as systemic hypertension, diabetes, coronary artery disease, and metabolic syndrome, which could result in an inaccurate underlying diagnosis.

PATHOLOGY
The Pulmonary Vasculature

PAH predominantly affects the small resistance pulmonary arteries, characterized by intimal hyperplasia, medial hypertrophy, adventitial proliferation, in situ thrombosis, and inflammation (**Fig. 1**).[24] Plexiform arteriopathy, which refers to capillarylike, angioproliferative vascular channels within the lumina of small muscular arteries, is the pathognomonic lesion of PAH.[24] Plexiform lesions often appear at branch points, frequently have fibrin thrombi within the lumen, and have varying channel diameter, giving them a disordered appearance.

The Right Ventricle

The chronic elevation in right ventricle (RV) afterload due to increased PVR induces right ventricular hypertrophy (RVH), which can be either adaptive or maladaptive (**Fig. 2**). Adaptive RVH, characterized by concentric hypertrophy with minimal eccentric dilatation and fibrosis, maintains normal ejection fraction, cardiac output, and filling pressures.[24] However, maladaptive RVH shows eccentric dilatation, increased fibrosis, and capillary rarefaction with reduction in ejection fraction and cardiac output and elevation in filling pressures.[24,25] At a metabolic level, maladaptive RVH is characterized by increased aerobic glycolysis, fatty acid oxidation, and glutaminolysis.[26] In addition, maladaptive RVH is associated with increased sympathetic activation and downregulation of α, β, and dopaminergic receptors in myocytes of the RV.[27] Furthermore, maladaptive RVH is associated with increased beta-myosin heavy chains (hypo contractile) and decreased alpha-myosin heavy chains (hyper contractile) similar to the fetal heart.[28] Some patients, especially those with congenital heart disease–associated PAH, remain stable with

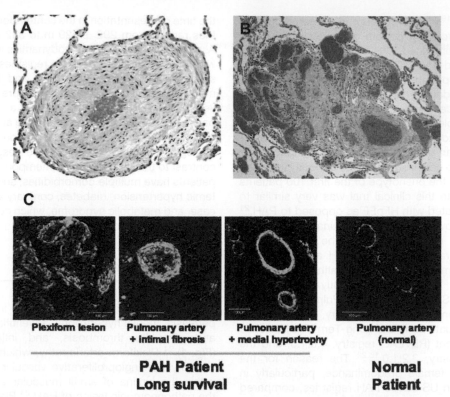

Fig. 1. Examples of pathologic changes with medial hypertrophy of pulmonary arteriole (*A*) and plexiform lesion (*B*) of hematoxylin-eosin stained lung sections at 20× magnification. (*C*) Smooth muscle actin is shown in green in to highlight vascular proliferation in PAH. (*Adapted from* Rich S, Pogoriler J, Husain AN, et al. Long-term effects of epoprostenol on the pulmonary vasculature in idiopathic pulmonary arterial hypertension. Chest 2010;138(5):1236; with permission.)

adaptive RVH for a prolonged period.[29,30] However, certain patients with PAH, specifically those with scleroderma-associated PAH, develop maladaptive RVH relatively early, leading to RV failure and death.[31] The mechanisms that mediate the switch from adaptive, compensatory hypertrophy of the RV to maladaptive RV dilatation and ultimately RV failure are unclear and are under investigation.[27,32] More research is needed to answer these questions, as long-term outcomes in PAH are largely determined by the response of the RV to the increased afterload.[33]

Adaptive RVH   Maladaptive RVH

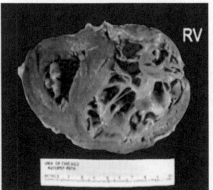

Fig. 2. Examples of adaptive and maladaptive RV remodeling in PAH. (*Adapted from* Rich S, Pogoriler J, Husain AN, et al. Long-term effects of epoprostenol on the pulmonary vasculature in idiopathic pulmonary arterial hypertension. Chest 2010;138(5):1237; with permission.)

PATHOGENESIS

Pulmonary Vascular Dysfunction

The pathogenesis of PAH likely involves multiple pathways rather than a single mechanism. There is an imbalance of vasoconstricting and vasodilating substances in the small pulmonary arteries. Increased production of the vasoconstrictors thromboxane, endothelin, and serotonin and reduced synthesis of vasodilators prostacyclin, nitric oxide, and vasoactive intestinal polypeptide were observed in patients with PAH.[1] This imbalance in favor of vasoconstrictors causes small pulmonary artery vasoconstriction. The change in abundance of these vasoactive chemicals has important implications beyond simply vasoactivity, as thromboxane induces platelet proliferation, prostacyclin inhibits smooth muscle proliferation and has antiplatelet properties, nitric oxide inhibits smooth muscle proliferation and inhibits platelet activation, and endothelin induces smooth muscle cell proliferation.[1] **Fig. 3** summarizes the known mechanisms that contribute to pulmonary vascular dysfunction in PAH.

Pulmonary Vascular Proliferation

There are changes in multiple pathways in the pulmonary artery smooth muscle cells that promote cellular replication and decreased apoptosis that contribute to the pulmonary vascular proliferation. Inappropriate activation of transcription factors hypoxia inducible factor (HIF)-1 alpha and nuclear factor of activated T-cells, decreased expression of voltage-gated potassium channels (eg, Kv1.5 and Kv2.1), increased expression of the antiapoptotic protein survivin, and increased expression of transient receptor potential channels (TRPC 6), which leads to calcium overload, are all pathways that promote smooth muscle propagation.[34] Finally, there is strong evidence that imbalance of mitochondrial fission and fusion leading to

excessive mitochondrial fission, also stimulates pulmonary arterial smooth muscle proliferation.[35] Thus, multiple pathways converge to contribute to excessive pulmonary arterial smooth muscle proliferation in PAH (**Fig. 4**).

Extracellular Matrix Remodeling

There is emerging evidence that extracellular matrix remodeling may be one of the inciting events in PAH pathophysiology. First, in the monocrotaline-induced rat PH model, fragmentation of the internal elastic lamina in the hilar pulmonary arteries occurs 2 days after monocrotaline injection, and 14 days before pulmonary artery smooth muscle hypertrophy.[36] Disruption of the internal elastic lamina is associated with increased elastolytic activity of serine elastases and matrix metalloproteinases in this animal model. Similar findings were reported in animal models of chronic hypoxic PH.[37] Inhibition of serine elastases prevented development of PH in both these animal models, confirming the pathogenic role of extracellular matrix remodeling in distal pulmonary arterial smooth muscle proliferation.[37-40]

Inflammation

Pathologic examination of the pulmonary vasculature, both in animal models of PH and patients with PAH, showed inflammatory cell infiltration, suggesting inflammation might contribute to pulmonary vascular remodeling.[41] Further investigation of the role of inflammation in PH led to the observations that serum levels of inflammatory cytokines (interleukin [IL]-1β, IL2, IL-6, IL-8, IL-10, IL-12, and tumor necrosis factor-α) were elevated in patients with PAH,[42,43] and serum levels of IL-6, IL-8, IL-10, and IL-12 predicted survival in PAH.[43] IL-6 has been the most intensively studied inflammatory cytokine in PAH. Animal data supported a role of IL-6 in promoting PAH, as IL-6 knockout

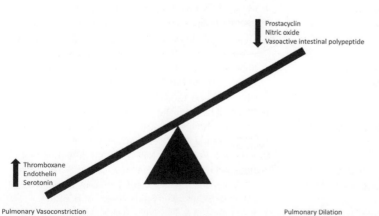

Prostacyclin
Nitric oxide
Vasoactive intestinal polypeptide

Thromboxane
Endothelin
Serotonin

Pulmonary Vasoconstriction

Pulmonary Dilation

Fig. 3. Schematic representation of imbalance of vasodilatory and vasoconstricting substances present in the pulmonary circulation in PAH leading to pulmonary vascular dysfunction in PAH.

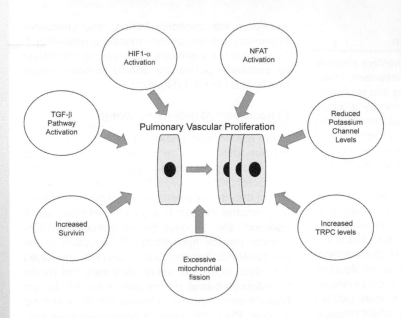

Fig. 4. Multiple pathways converge to induce pulmonary vascular proliferation in PAH.

mice were resistant to hypoxia-induced PH,[44] whereas overexpression of IL-6 induced PH.[45] Moreover, use of the IL-6 receptor antibody tocilizumab reduced the severity of PH in patients with Castleman disease,[46,47] providing further evidence that elevated IL-6 levels promote a more severe PAH phenotype.

RIGHT VENTRICULAR PATHOLOGIC CHANGES
Right Ventricular Metabolic Derangements

As with vascular remodeling, multiple pathways are implicated in RV dysfunction in PAH (**Fig. 5**). Work aimed at understanding the switch between adaptive and maladaptive RV remodeling has identified metabolic derangements as a likely

mediator. In particular, mitochondrial dysfunction marked by reduced oxidative metabolism[25] and ectopic glutaminolysis[48] has been shown to play a role in RV dysfunction in PAH.

- A shift from oxidative to anaerobic metabolism of glucose occurs in the RV in PAH. This can lead to an energy-starved state, as anaerobic metabolism of glucose produces less ATP than aerobic metabolism of glucose (2 ATP per glucose in anaerobic metabolism vs 36 ATP with coupled oxidative metabolism). To compensate for reduced metabolic efficacy of anaerobic glycolysis, glucose uptake by the RV is increased to generate more ATP.[49]

Fig. 5. Mechanisms that contribute to RV failure in PAH.

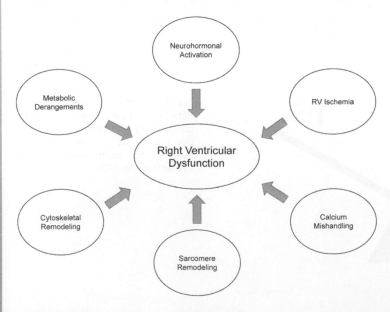

- Similar to cancer cell metabolism, there is normoxic activation of HIF-1 alpha (Warburg effect) in the RV in PAH, which activates pyruvate dehydrogenase kinase (PDK). Activation of PDK inhibits pyruvate dehydrogenase, the rate-limiting enzyme for aerobic glucose oxidation.[25]
- Activation of oxidative metabolism through inhibition of pyruvate dehydrogenase kinase using dichloroacetate improved RV function in animal models of PAH.[50,51]
- There is increased fatty acid oxidation in the RV in PAH. Inhibition of fatty acid oxidation, using either ranolazine or trimetazidine, led to a reciprocal increase in glucose oxidation and improved RV function (Randall cycle) in animal models of PH.[52]
- Glutaminolysis, metabolism of glutamine, a metabolic pathway that is usually detected only in cancer cells, was identified in the RV of animals with RV hypertrophy. Inhibition of glutaminolysis enhanced glucose oxidation and improved RV function and exercise capacity.[48]

Right Ventricular Ischemia

Another factor that contributes to maladaptive RV remodeling and metabolic changes is RV ischemia due to reduced right coronary artery epicardial flow and capillary rarefaction associated with PAH.

- In the normal RV, perfusion from the right coronary artery occurs during systole and diastole. However, in PAH, elevated RV systolic pressure minimizes the pressure differences between the right coronary artery and the aorta and thus reduces filling time (only during diastole as opposed to both systole and diastole) and RV perfusion.[53]
- Impaired angiogenesis demonstrated by reduced number of capillaries and intramuscular arterioles can also contribute to RV ischemia,[54] a phenotype often observed in scleroderma-associated PAH. Patients with scleroderma typically display maladaptive RV remodeling,[31] providing more evidence that relative RV ischemia contributes to RV failure in PAH.

Right Ventricular Calcium Mishandling

Although the cellular mechanisms of left ventricular dysfunction has been extensively studied, the understanding of the causes of RV dysfunction in PAH has lagged behind. However, recent data have emerged that suggest calcium mishandling contributes to RV dysfunction in PAH.

- In a canine model of PH caused by PA banding, decreased amounts of SERCA-2a and phosphorylated phospholamban, which was relative to the degree of increased afterload, were observed.[55]
- In the monocrotaline rat model, decreased levels of SERCA-2a protein and mRNA levels of phospholamban and ryanodine receptor were documented in the RV.[56]
- In the monocrotaline rat model, calcium transients were noted to be smaller with slower kinetics to peak and decay. This was associated with a reduction in L-type calcium-channel protein levels.[57]

Sarcomere Remodeling

As observed in cardiomyocyte dysfunction in the left ventricle, there are derangements of the sarcomeric proteins in the RV in PAH.

- Myosin isoform switches: Increased β-myosin heavy chain mRNA and decreased α-myosin heavy chain mRNA was documented in samples of patients with PAH and RV failure.[28] Animal models with similar myosin isoform switching had reduced contractility[58] likely due to different ATPase activities of the α-myosin and β-myosin heavy chains.
- Change in actin isoforms: A 10-fold increase in the amount of skeletal muscle α-actin mRNA in the right ventricle was found in the high-altitude calf model of PH.[59] The functional consequences of this change remain unknown.

Cytoskeletal Remodeling

Increased stabilization and subsequent proliferation of the microtubule cytoskeleton was documented in preclinical models of PH. However, there are mixed results on the pathologic consequences of microtubule proliferation in the RV.

- Microtubule stabilization and proliferation was documented in the PA-banded feline model. Microtubule depolymerization normalized cardiac contractility in isolated cardiomyocytes.[60,61]
- The rat monocrotaline PAH model also showed increased microtubules, but colchicine-induced microtubule depolymerization did not enhance contractility in isolated cardiomyocytes.[62]

GENETIC CAUSES OF PULMONARY ARTERIAL HYPERTENSION

PAH also can be inherited. Approximately, 10% of patients have hereditable PAH, which is outlined as follows.

- Transforming growth factor beta (TGF-ß) pathway mutations
  - Bone morphogenetic protein receptor (BMPR2): Regulates vascular smooth muscle cell growth by activating the intracellular pathways of SMAD and LIM kinase. Loss of function mutation of the *BMPR2* gene leads to decreased activation of SMAD, ultimately leading to increased proliferation of pulmonary artery smooth muscle cells.[63]
  - Activin receptor-like kinase 1: Receptor for TGF-β superfamily of ligands with mutations associated with PAH. Activation of this receptor leads to increased proliferation of pulmonary artery smooth muscle cells.[64,65]
  - Endoglin: Membrane-bound TGF-β receptor, which when activated induces cellular replication.[65]
- Caveolin-1: A membrane protein that forms caveolae, which are flask-shaped invaginations of the plasma membrane. Caveolae regulates membrane trafficking, cell signaling, cholesterol homeostasis, and mechanotransduction.[66]
- KCNK3: Two-pore potassium channel expressed in pulmonary artery smooth muscle cells. This potassium channel modulates resting membrane potential, pulmonary vascular tone, and hypoxic pulmonary vasoconstriction.[67]

SUMMARY

Although our knowledge about the epidemiology and pathophysiology of PAH has increased greatly in the past 20 years, PAH continues to be a debilitating disease with poor survival and high economic burden. There are still many unanswered questions that will need to be investigated to reduce symptomatic burden and promote patient survival in the future.

REFERENCES

1. Farber HW, Loscalzo J. Pulmonary arterial hypertension. N Engl J Med 2004;351(16):1655–65.
2. Rich S, Dantzker DR, Ayres SM, et al. Primary pulmonary hypertension. A national prospective study. Ann Intern Med 1987;107(2):216–23.
3. D'Alonzo GE, Barst RJ, Ayres SM, et al. Survival in patients with primary pulmonary hypertension. Results from a national prospective registry. Ann Intern Med 1991;115(5):343–9.
4. Thenappan T, Shah SJ, Rich S, et al. Survival in pulmonary arterial hypertension: a reappraisal of the NIH risk stratification equation. Eur Respir J 2010; 35(5):1079–87.
5. Galiè N, Corris PA, Frost A, et al. Updated treatment algorithm of pulmonary arterial hypertension. J Am Coll Cardiol 2013;62(25 Suppl):D60–72.
6. Humbert M, Sitbon O, Chaouat A, et al. Pulmonary arterial hypertension in France: results from a national registry. Am J Respir Crit Care Med 2006; 173(9):1023–30.
7. Thenappan T, Shah SJ, Rich S, et al. A USA-based registry for pulmonary arterial hypertension: 1982-2006. Eur Respir J 2007;30(6):1103–10.
8. Badesch DB, Raskob GE, Elliott CG, et al. Pulmonary arterial hypertension: baseline characteristics from the REVEAL registry. Chest 2010;137(2):376–87.
9. Ling Y, Johnson MK, Kiely DG, et al. Changing demographics, epidemiology, and survival of incident pulmonary arterial hypertension: results from the pulmonary hypertension registry of the United Kingdom and Ireland. Am J Respir Crit Care Med 2012;186(8):790–6.
10. Escribano-Subias P, Blanco I, López-Meseguer M, et al. Survival in pulmonary hypertension in Spain: insights from the Spanish registry. Eur Respir J 2012;40(3):596–603.
11. Hoeper MM, Huscher D, Ghofrani HA, et al. Elderly patients diagnosed with idiopathic pulmonary arterial hypertension: results from the COMPERA registry. Int J Cardiol 2013;168(2):871–80.
12. Zhang R, Dai LZ, Xie WP, et al. Survival of Chinese patients with pulmonary arterial hypertension in the modern treatment era. Chest 2011;140(2):301–9.
13. Peacock AJ, Murphy NF, McMurray JJ, et al. An epidemiological study of pulmonary arterial hypertension. Eur Respir J 2007;30(1):104–9.
14. Jing ZC, Xu XQ, Han ZY, et al. Registry and survival study in Chinese patients with idiopathic and familial pulmonary arterial hypertension. Chest 2007;132(2): 373–9.
15. Kane GC, Maradit-Kremers H, Slusser JP, et al. Integration of clinical and hemodynamic parameters in the prediction of long-term survival in patients with pulmonary arterial hypertension. Chest 2011; 139(6):1285–93.
16. Frost AE, Badesch DB, Barst RJ, et al. The changing picture of patients with pulmonary arterial hypertension in the United States: how REVEAL differs from historic and non-US contemporary registries. Chest 2011;139(1):128–37.
17. Halpern SD, Taichman DB. Misclassification of pulmonary hypertension due to reliance on pulmonary capillary wedge pressure rather than left ventricular end-diastolic pressure. Chest 2009;136(1):37–43.

18. Thenappan T, Shah SJ, Gomberg-Maitland M, et al. Clinical characteristics of pulmonary hypertension in patients with heart failure and preserved ejection fraction. Circ Heart Fail 2011;4(3):257–65.

19. Ryan JJ, Rich JD, Thiruvoipati T, et al. Current practice for determining pulmonary capillary wedge pressure predisposes to serious errors in the classification of patients with pulmonary hypertension. Am Heart J 2012;163(4):589–94.

20. Kovacs G, Avian A, Pienn M, et al. Reading pulmonary vascular pressure tracings. How to handle the problems of zero leveling and respiratory swings. Am J Respir Crit Care Med 2014;190(3):252–7.

21. Galiè N, Barberà JA, Frost AE, et al. Initial use of ambrisentan plus tadalafil in pulmonary arterial hypertension. N Engl J Med 2015;373(9):834–44.

22. McGoon MD, Benza RL, Escribano-Subias P, et al. Pulmonary arterial hypertension: epidemiology and registries. J Am Coll Cardiol 2013;62(25 Suppl):D51–9.

23. Brown LM, Chen H, Halpern S, et al. Delay in recognition of pulmonary arterial hypertension: factors identified from the REVEAL Registry. Chest 2011;140(1):19–26.

24. Rich S, Pogoriler J, Husain AN, et al. Long-term effects of epoprostenol on the pulmonary vasculature in idiopathic pulmonary arterial hypertension. Chest 2010;138(5):1234–9.

25. Ryan JJ, Archer SL. The right ventricle in pulmonary arterial hypertension: disorders of metabolism, angiogenesis and adrenergic signaling in right ventricular failure. Circ Res 2014;115(1):176–88.

26. Archer SL, Fang YH, Ryan JJ, et al. Metabolism and bioenergetics in the right ventricle and pulmonary vasculature in pulmonary hypertension. Pulm Circ 2013;3(1):144–52.

27. Piao L, Fang YH, Parikh KS, et al. GRK2-mediated inhibition of adrenergic and dopaminergic signaling in right ventricular hypertrophy: therapeutic implications in pulmonary hypertension. Circulation 2012;126(24):2859–69.

28. Lowes BD, Minobe W, Abraham WT, et al. Changes in gene expression in the intact human heart. Downregulation of alpha-myosin heavy chain in hypertrophied, failing ventricular myocardium. J Clin Invest 1997;100(9):2315–24.

29. Reddy S, Bernstein D. Molecular mechanisms of right ventricular failure. Circulation 2015;132(18):1734–42.

30. Vonk-Noordegraaf A, Haddad F, Chin KM, et al. Right heart adaptation to pulmonary arterial hypertension: physiology and pathobiology. J Am Coll Cardiol 2013;62(25 Suppl):D22–33.

31. Tedford RJ, Mudd JO, Girgis RE, et al. Right ventricular dysfunction in systemic sclerosis-associated pulmonary arterial hypertension. Circ Heart Fail 2013;6(5):953–63.

32. Drake JI, Gomez-Arroyo J, Dumur CI, et al. Chronic carvedilol treatment partially reverses the right ventricular failure transcriptional profile in experimental pulmonary hypertension. Physiol Genomics 2013;45(12):449–61.

33. van de Veerdonk MC, Kind T, Marcus JT, et al. Progressive right ventricular dysfunction in patients with pulmonary arterial hypertension responding to therapy. J Am Coll Cardiol 2011;58(24):2511–9.

34. Tuder RM, Archer SL, Dorfmüller P, et al. Relevant issues in the pathology and pathobiology of pulmonary hypertension. J Am Coll Cardiol 2013;62(25 Suppl):D4–12.

35. Archer SL. Mitochondrial dynamics–mitochondrial fission and fusion in human diseases. N Engl J Med 2013;369(23):2236–51.

36. Todorovich-Hunter L, Dodo H, Ye C, et al. Increased pulmonary artery elastolytic activity in adult rats with monocrotaline-induced progressive hypertensive pulmonary vascular disease compared with infant rats with nonprogressive disease. Am Rev Respir Dis 1992;146(1):213–23.

37. Maruyama K, Ye CL, Woo M, et al. Chronic hypoxic pulmonary hypertension in rats and increased elastolytic activity. Am J Physiol 1991;261(6 Pt 2):H1716–26.

38. Zaidi SH, You XM, Ciura S, et al. Overexpression of the serine elastase inhibitor elafin protects transgenic mice from hypoxic pulmonary hypertension. Circulation 2002;105(4):516–21.

39. Ilkiw R, Todorovich-Hunter L, Maruyama K, et al. SC-39026, a serine elastase inhibitor, prevents muscularization of peripheral arteries, suggesting a mechanism of monocrotaline-induced pulmonary hypertension in rats. Circ Res 1989;64(4):814–25.

40. Ye CL, Rabinovitch M. Inhibition of elastolysis by SC-37698 reduces development and progression of monocrotaline pulmonary hypertension. Am J Physiol 1991;261(4 Pt 2):H1255–67.

41. Hassoun PM, Mouthon L, Barberà JA, et al. Inflammation, growth factors, and pulmonary vascular remodeling. J Am Coll Cardiol 2009;54(1 Suppl):S10–9.

42. Humbert M, Monti G, Brenot F, et al. Increased interleukin-1 and interleukin-6 serum concentrations in severe primary pulmonary hypertension. Am J Respir Crit Care Med 1995;151(5):1628–31.

43. Soon E, Holmes AM, Treacy CM, et al. Elevated levels of inflammatory cytokines predict survival in idiopathic and familial pulmonary arterial hypertension. Circulation 2010;122(9):920–7.

44. Savale L, Tu L, Rideau D, et al. Impact of interleukin-6 on hypoxia-induced pulmonary hypertension and lung inflammation in mice. Respir Res 2009;10:6.

45. Steiner MK, Syrkina OL, Kolliputi N, et al. Interleukin-6 overexpression induces pulmonary hypertension. Circ Res 2009;104(2):236–44 [28p following 244].

46. Taniguchi K, Shimazaki C, Fujimoto Y, et al. Tocilizumab is effective for pulmonary hypertension associated with multicentric Castleman's disease. Int J Hematol 2009;90(1):99–102.

47. Arita Y, Sakata Y, Sudo T, et al. The efficacy of tocilizumab in a patient with pulmonary arterial hypertension associated with Castleman's disease. Heart Vessels 2010;25(5):444–7.

48. Piao L, Fang YH, Parikh K, et al. Cardiac glutaminolysis: a maladaptive cancer metabolism pathway in the right ventricle in pulmonary hypertension. J Mol Med (Berl) 2013;91(10):1185–97.

49. Ryan JJ, Huston J, Kutty S, et al. Right ventricular adaptation and failure in pulmonary arterial hypertension. Can J Cardiol 2015;31(4):391–406.

50. McMurtry MS, Bonnet S, Wu X, et al. Dichloroacetate prevents and reverses pulmonary hypertension by inducing pulmonary artery smooth muscle cell apoptosis. Circ Res 2004;95(8):830–40.

51. Michelakis ED, McMurtry MS, Wu XC, et al. Dichloroacetate, a metabolic modulator, prevents and reverses chronic hypoxic pulmonary hypertension in rats: role of increased expression and activity of voltage-gated potassium channels. Circulation 2002;105(2):244–50.

52. Fang YH, Piao L, Hong Z, et al. Therapeutic inhibition of fatty acid oxidation in right ventricular hypertrophy: exploiting Randle's cycle. J Mol Med (Berl) 2012;90(1):31–43.

53. van Wolferen SA, Marcus JT, Westerhof N, et al. Right coronary artery flow impairment in patients with pulmonary hypertension. Eur Heart J 2008; 29(1):120–7.

54. Bogaard HJ, Natarajan R, Henderson SC, et al. Chronic pulmonary artery pressure elevation is insufficient to explain right heart failure. Circulation 2009;120(20):1951–60.

55. Moon MR, Aziz A, Lee AM, et al. Differential calcium handling in two canine models of right ventricular pressure overload. J Surg Res 2012;178(2):554–62.

56. Kögler H, Hartmann O, Leineweber K, et al. Mechanical load-dependent regulation of gene expression in monocrotaline-induced right ventricular hypertrophy in the rat. Circ Res 2003;93(3):230–7.

57. Xie YP, Chen B, Sanders P, et al. Sildenafil prevents and reverses transverse-tubule remodeling and Ca(2+) handling dysfunction in right ventricle failure induced by pulmonary artery hypertension. Hypertension 2012;59(2):355–62.

58. Herron TJ, McDonald KS. Small amounts of alpha-myosin heavy chain isoform expression significantly increase power output of rat cardiac myocyte fragments. Circ Res 2002;90(11):1150–2.

59. Bakerman PR, Stenmark KR, Fisher JH. Alpha-skeletal actin messenger RNA increases in acute right ventricular hypertrophy. Am J Physiol 1990;258(4 Pt 1):L173–8.

60. Tsutsui H, Ishihara K, Cooper G. Cytoskeletal role in the contractile dysfunction of hypertrophied myocardium. Science 1993;260(5108):682–7.

61. Tsutsui H, Tagawa H, Kent RL, et al. Role of microtubules in contractile dysfunction of hypertrophied cardiocytes. Circulation 1994;90(1):533–55.

62. Stones R, Benoist D, Peckham M, et al. Microtubule proliferation in right ventricular myocytes of rats with monocrotaline-induced pulmonary hypertension. J Mol Cell Cardiol 2013;56:91–6.

63. Best DH, Austin ED, Chung WK, et al. Genetics of pulmonary hypertension. Curr Opin Cardiol 2014; 29(6):520–7.

64. Abdalla SA, Gallione CJ, Barst RJ, et al. Primary pulmonary hypertension in families with hereditary haemorrhagic telangiectasia. Eur Respir J 2004;23(3): 373–7.

65. Harrison RE, Flanagan JA, Sankelo M, et al. Molecular and functional analysis identifies ALK-1 as the predominant cause of pulmonary hypertension related to hereditary haemorrhagic telangiectasia. J Med Genet 2003;40(12):865–71.

66. Austin ED, Ma L, LeDuc C, et al. Whole exome sequencing to identify a novel gene (caveolin-1) associated with human pulmonary arterial hypertension. Circ Cardiovasc Genet 2012;5(3): 336–43.

67. Ma L, Chung WK. The genetic basis of pulmonary arterial hypertension. Hum Genet 2014;133(5): 471–9.

Pulmonary Arterial Hypertension
Diagnosis and Treatment

Christopher F. Barnett, MD, MPH[a,b], Paulino Alvarez, MD[c],
Myung H. Park, MD[d],*

KEYWORDS

- Pulmonary arterial hypertension • Echocardiography • Right heart catheterization • Prostacyclin
- Phosphodiesterase inhibitor • Endothelin antagonist

KEY POINTS

- Pulmonary arterial hypertension is a rapidly progressive disease of the pulmonary circulation; despite improvements in available treatments, morbidity and mortality remains high.
- The time from symptom onset to diagnosis in pulmonary arterial hypertension is often long; this can delay initiation of treatment and contribute to worse outcomes.
- Echocardiography is often the initial test for screening patients at increased risk of pulmonary arterial hypertension or patients with symptoms suggestive of pulmonary arterial hypertension.
- Right heart catheterization is mandatory in all patients with possible pulmonary arterial hypertension to confirm the diagnosis, determine disease severity, and guide selection of initial therapy.
- Treatments for pulmonary arterial hypertension are complex and best accomplished with a multidisciplinary team, the rationale for guideline recommendation for close collaboration with a center with expertise in the diagnosis and management of pulmonary hypertension.

 Video content accompanies this article at http://www.cardiology.theclinics.com.

INTRODUCTION

Among healthy adults, a normal resting mean pulmonary artery pressure (mPAP) is 14 ± 3.3 mm Hg with a maximum value of 20.6 mm Hg. Pulmonary hypertension (PH) is the term used to describe the finding of a mPAP ≥ 25 mm Hg regardless of the underlying cause.

In contrast, pulmonary arterial hypertension (PAH) is a specific disease characterized by pathologic pulmonary vascular remodeling. This is referred to as idiopathic PAH (IPAH) for patients without an underlying cause; PAH can also be associated in the setting of a systemic condition such as human immunodeficiency virus (HIV) infection, systemic sclerosis (SSc), portal hypertension, and exposure to toxins and drugs. Hemodynamically, PAH is defined by a mPAP ≥ 25 mm Hg with normal left heart filling pressures defined as a pulmonary artery wedge pressure (PAWP) <15 mm Hg. In untreated PAH, increased

[a] Medstar Heart and Vascular Institute, 110 Irving Street Northwest Washington, DC 20010, USA; [b] Critical Care Medicine Department, National Institutes of Health, 10 Center Drive, Room 2C145, Bethesda, MD 20892, USA; [c] Department of Cardiology, Methodist DeBakey Heart & Vascular Center, Houston Methodist Hospital, 6550 Fannin Street, Smith Tower, Suite 1901, Houston, TX 77030, USA; [d] Division of Heart Failure and Transplant, Department of Cardiology, Methodist DeBakey Heart & Vascular Center, Houston Methodist Hospital, 6550 Fannin Street, Smith Tower, Suite 1901, Houston, TX 77030, USA
* Corresponding author.
E-mail address: mhpark@houstonmethodist.org

Cardiol Clin 34 (2016) 375–389
http://dx.doi.org/10.1016/j.ccl.2016.04.006
0733-8651/16/$ – see front matter © 2016 Elsevier Inc. All rights reserved.

right ventricular (RV) afterload rapidly leads to right ventricular failure and death.

This review discusses the comprehensive diagnostic assessment necessary to evaluate patients with suspected PAH and the currently recommended approaches for treatment of PAH.

COLLABORATIVE CARE WITH A PULMONARY HYPERTENSION REFERRAL CENTER

Current guidelines recommend comprehensive diagnostic testing and early aggressive treatment of PAH; however, recent data show that management for many patients is not optimal. In one study of patients referred to PH expert centers, 61% of patients had advanced disease with New York Heart Association (NYHA) class III or IV symptoms, 33% had an incorrect diagnosis, and 57% were receiving an incorrect medication.[1] In another report among patients with PAH, of which 78% were receiving PAH therapy, a complete diagnostic evaluation had been performed in only 6% of patients, and only 7% of patients treated with calcium channel blockers met criteria.[2] To address these deficiencies and improve PAH care and patient outcomes, early referral to PH specialty centers and collaborative care with community providers are recommended.

DIAGNOSIS

The goals of the diagnostic evaluation are to (1) detect elevated PAP or other findings that suggest PH is present, (2) confirm the diagnosis via right heart catheterization (RHC) and determine the etiology of PH, and (3) evaluate for the presence of high-risk features to aide in the choice of initial therapy. In some patients, the cause of PH is clearly evident; however, in many patients, differentiating PAH from the more common PH owing to left heart disease (PH-LHD) and PH lung disease can present a significant diagnostic challenge. The diagnostic approach to patients with suspected PAH is described in **Fig. 1**.

Screening

Screening is recommended in select patients with risk factors for PAH (**Table 1**). Screening in SSc is recommended using echocardiographic and pulmonary function tests criteria including diffusion capacity (DLCO).[3] Use of the multimodal DETECT algorithm for PAH screening in SSc patients was recently reported to be 96% sensitive for PAH compared with 71% for standard approaches to screening.[4]

Screening or symptom-triggered echocardiography should be considered in patients with a genetic predisposition to PAH, sickle cell disease, HIV, a history of congenital heart disease, anorexigen use, or liver disease.[5]

General Approach

Symptoms of PAH are nonspecific, which contributes to the delay in diagnosis. Symptoms can be classified as:

- Early
  - Exercise limitation due to fatigues or dyspnea
- Late
  - Related to low cardiac output and right ventricular failure: edema, ascites, dyspnea at rest, cyanosis and syncope
  - Related to enlargement of the pulmonary artery: hoarseness, angina due to coronary artery compression

A history of connective tissue disease (CTD), HIV, liver disease, and methamphetamine use suggests PAH, whereas a history of significant LHD or lung disease makes PAH less likely. Clinical characteristics including advanced age, hypertension, atrial fibrillation, and diabetes suggest a diagnosis of heart failure with preserved ejection fraction (HFpEF), which is a common cause of PH.

Physical examination may find signs of right ventricular failure, including jugular venous distention, right ventricular third heart sound or heave, and cool and edematous lower extremities. Joint and skin findings suggestive of CTD or stigmata of liver disease may point to PAH, whereas presence of rales or left-sided heart murmurs suggest PH-LHD or PH from lung disease.

Laboratory tests should include CTD and HIV serologies. Urine testing for methamphetamine and cocaine should also be considered. Elevated brain natriuretic peptide levels provide useful prognostic information in PAH patients.

Findings of right atrial abnormality or right ventricular hypertrophy may be present on electrocardiograms in advanced stages; however, normal electrocardiogram does not rule out PAH. Abnormalities of the left atrial and ventricle or atrial fibrillation are suggestive of PH-LHD (**Fig. 2**).[6]

Classic chest radiograph findings in patients with PAH occur late in the disease and include prominence of the main pulmonary arteries and a reduction in the number of peripheral blood vessels and RV enlargement in lateral image (see **Fig. 2**).[6]

Echocardiography

Echocardiography is often the first test performed when PAH is suspected and is used to monitor disease progression and treatment effects. An

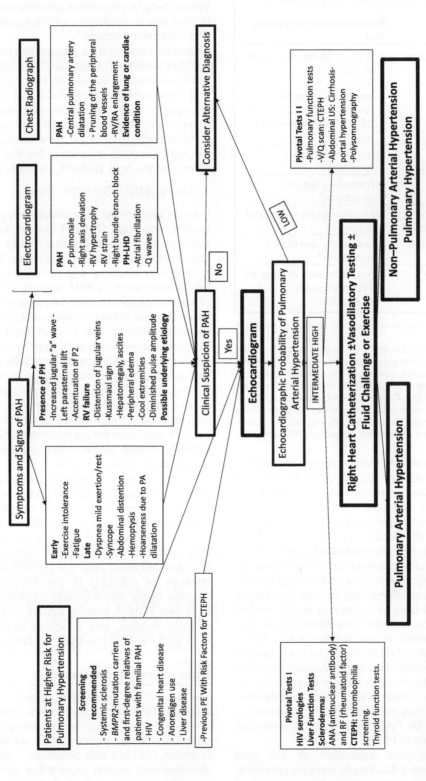

Fig. 1. Diagnostic approach to patients in whom PAH is suspected.

Table 1
Screening for PAH in high-risk populations

Population	Recommended Screening Test
Systemic sclerosis	• Annual spirometry with DLCO • Annual echocardiography • Annual evaluation using DETECT algorithm (96% sensitive)
Genetic predisposition	Echocardiogram for symptoms[a]
HIV	Echocardiogram for symptoms[a]
Congenital or repaired shunt	Echocardiogram at time of diagnosis
Anorexigen use	Echocardiogram for symptoms[a]
Liver disease	Echocardiogram at time of liver transplant evaluation

[a] Symptoms of exertional dyspnea, edema, presyncope, syncope.

Adapted from McLaughlin VV, Archer SL, Badesch DB, et al. ACCF/AHA 2009 expert consensus document on pulmonary hypertension: a report of the American College of Cardiology Foundation Task Force on Expert Consensus Documents and the American Heart Association: developed in collaboration with the American College of Chest Physicians, American Thoracic Society, Inc., and the Pulmonary Hypertension Association. Circulation 2009;119:2263.

integrative approach that combines the pulmonary artery systolic pressure (PASP), RV function, and other findings is recommended (**Table 2**).[7]

The PASP is estimated by combining the peak tricuspid regurgitant jet velocity (V) and the RA pressure (RAP) in the equation: PASP = $4(V^2)$+RAP. However, a tricuspid regurgitation jet adequate for analysis may not be present in up to 60% of patients depending on factors such as body habitus and the presence of parenchymal lung disease. Poor quality of the spectral Doppler signal may lead to over or underestimation of PASP. The PASP may be also be low secondary to low cardiac output in the setting of advanced RV failure. In one study, despite a reasonable correlation with invasively assessed PASP (r = 0.66; P<.001), 48% of 65 patients had echo estimated PASP at least 10 mm Hg different from the invasively measured PASP.[8] These errors in estimation of PASP may lead to important misclassification of PH.

Echocardiographic evaluation of the right ventricle is made difficult by its complex geometric shape and contractile motion. The presence of enlarged and hypertrophied right heart chambers and flattening or a D-shaped interventricular septum provide indirect evidence of PAH (**Fig. 3**, Videos 1–4). A pericardial effusion may be seen in PAH and is associated with advanced disease and increased mortality.[6]

Standard quantitative approaches to assess RV function have been described[9] (**Fig. 4**); however, each approach is subject to important technical and methodologic limitations, so the overall impression of an experienced echocardiographer is important. Measurement of the RV ejection fraction is not reliable because of the irregular shape of the right ventricle; however, the fractional area change of the right ventricle, defined by

$$FAC = (EDV-ESV)/EDV \times 100$$

may be determined. The tricuspid annular plane systolic excursion (TAPSE) is a measure of the distance the tricuspid annulus moves toward the right ventricular apex during systole. The TAPSE is simple to measure and provides useful prognostic information in PAH. Velocity of the motion of the tricuspid annulus can be measured by pulsed tissue Doppler of the tricuspid valve annulus and is abnormal if it is less than 10 cm/s. Both TAPSE and Doppler tissue imaging are limited by angle dependence of the measurement. Ventricular strain analysis using speckle tracking is appealing because it is angle independent and reproducible. Early studies have reported that RV strain is more useful than other echo parameters to predict outcomes in patients with heart failure; however, further investigation is needed before routine assessment of RV strain can be recommended.

Echocardiographic findings of reduced ejection fraction or valvular heart disease are generally readily detected and suggest a diagnosis of PH-LHD. Detecting HFpEF is more difficult, but a diagnosis of HFpEF should be considered in patients with elevated PASP, normal ejection fraction (EF), and left heart chamber abnormalities.[10] The absence of notching in the RV outflow tract Doppler signal also supports a diagnosis of PH-LHD over PAH. A scoring system that integrates multiple findings and is useful to differentiate PAH from PH-LHD has been described.[11]

Right Heart Catheterization

The requirement for invasive hemodynamic testing with RHC for definitive diagnosis in patients evaluated for PAH is supported universally in all PAH guidelines. When performed by an experienced operator, RHC is a safe procedure[12] and noninvasive methods cannot provide the complete and accurate measurements of all of the hemodynamic parameters required for correct diagnosis of PAH.

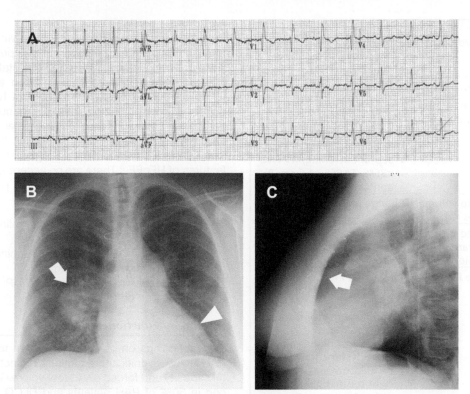

Fig. 2. Typical electrocardiogram and chest radiograph findings in PAH. Electrocardiogram shows right axis deviation, P wave in lead II >2.5 mm, qR pattern in V1, R/S >1 in V1, ST depression in the anterior precordial leads (*A*). Chest radiograph shows pulmonary artery dilatation (*arrow*), pruning of the peripheral pulmonary vessels, and an elevated apex in the posterior-anterior projection (*arrowhead*) (*B*). Obliteration of the retrosternal space secondary to RV enlargement is seen in the in the lateral projection (*arrow*) (*C*).

Expert recommendations for performing RHC have been published.[3] Close attention should be paid to ensure proper leveling and zeroing of transducers. The transducer should be zeroed at the level of the left atrium (midthoracic line in supine patient halfway between the anterior sternum and the bed surface), and transducer position should be documented. An appropriate response on the monitor to vertical movement of the catheter and to a rapid flush test ensure that the catheter system is adequately pressurized and no air bubbles are present. All waveforms should be critically evaluated to ensure that they are of high quality, and all pressures should be determined at end expiration to minimize the effects of intrathoracic pressure variation on the measurement.

A complete hemodynamic assessment includes measurement of.

- Right atrial pressure
- Right ventricular pressure (systolic, diastolic)
- Pulmonary artery pressure (systolic, diastolic, mean)
- Pulmonary artery wedge pressure
- Cardiac output and cardiac index

The Fick cardiac output formula assumes a basal oxygen consumption of 125 mL of oxygen per minute per square meter, a value that is usually not accurate in patients with PAH. The thermodilution cardiac output, when measured in triplicate and injected during end expiration, remains valid in most settings, even in that of low cardiac output and severe tricuspid regurgitation.[13]

The PAWP is used to estimate left ventricular end diastolic pressure (LVEDP). Incorrect determination of the PAWP may be secondary to errors including:

- Improper transducer position
- Waveform dampening
- Incompletely wedged catheter
- Measurement that is not at end expiration
- Use of the electronic mean obtained from the computer monitor

The oxygen saturation of a blood sample withdrawn with the catheter in the wedge position should closely approximate the systemic arterial saturation. Measurement performed manually on pressure tracings at end expiration is most tightly

Table 2
Echocardiographic assessment in PAH

Task	Method
Estimate PASP	PASP = $4V^2$+ RAP
Evaluate RV size and function	• RV>LV, RV shares apex with LV • RV end diastolic wall thickness >5 mm • Septal flattening, RV FAC <35%, TAPSE <1.6 cm, RV annular velocity <10 cm/s
Estimate volume status	Change in IVC diameter
Evaluate for pericardial effusion	Presence of pericardial effusion is a poor prognostic sign
Exclude PH-LHD	• Reduced EF • Mitral or aortic valve disease • Bubble study for intracardiac shunt • Grade 2 or higher diastolic dysfunction • LA enlargement, left to right septal bowing, E/A ratio >1.2, lateral E/e' >11, lateral e'<8 cm/s • RVOT pulse wave Doppler with notching

Abbreviations: FAC, fraction area change; IVC, inferior vena cava; LV, left ventricle; RVOT, right ventricular outflow tract; V, tricuspid regurgitant jet velocity.

correlated with the LVEDP. Measurement of the LVEDP should be performed whenever a reliable PAWP tracing cannot be obtained or the value of the PAWP is inconsistent with the expected value based on the clinical picture.[14]

Vasoreactivity testing

Vasoreactivity testing is useful for identifying the small number of patients who can be successfully treated with high-dose calcium channel blockers. Guidelines for vasoreactivity testing include:

- Testing is recommended for IPAH only.
- Agents used include inhaled nitric oxide, intravenous epoprostenol, or intravenous adenosine (**Table 3**).
- *Responsive* is defined as decrease in mPAP by >10 mm Hg to less than 40 mm Hg with no decrease in cardiac output or increase in PAWP.
- Development of pulmonary edema raises suspicion for the presence of pulmonary veno-occlusive disease, pulmonary capillary hemangiomatosis, or LHD.

Provocative testing

Patients with PAH generally present with symptoms during exertion. However, RHC is performed while patients are lying still in a fasting state, often after sedating medications have been administered, and only records a snapshot of hemodynamics at one moment in time. Recent guidelines recommend measurement of PAWP after provocative testing to uncover hemodynamic abnormalities consistent with LHD in patients with clinical features of HFpEF.[3] There are no accepted guidelines for provocative maneuvers but protocols generally call for:

- Fluid challenge 500 mL of normal saline over 5 to 10 minutes
- *OR* Exercise stress using a supine cycle ergometer or by lifting weights
- *AND* Repeat measurement of PAP, PAWP, and cardiac output

Pulmonary Function Tests

Typical findings on pulmonary function testing in PAH include significant reductions in functional vital capacity and forced expiratory volume in 1 second in 50% of PAH patients and DLCO in more than 75% of patients.[15] A low DLCO less than 60% is associated with PAH. Most often the forced expiratory volume in 1 second/functional vital capacity ratio in PAH is consistent with a restrictive ventilatory defect. Obstructive defects are less common and should prompt additional investigation for parenchymal lung disease.

Overnight Pulse Oximetry and Polysomnography

Nocturnal desaturation is common among patients with PAH and may increase PAP through hypoxic pulmonary vasoconstriction. Patients should be screened with overnight oximetry and supplemental oxygen prescribed as needed.[16] Sleep-disordered breathing may contribute to increased PAP and, if suspected, should be evaluated and treated.

Ventilation Perfusion Lung Scan

Ventilation perfusion lung scanning is required to exclude the diagnosis of chronic thromboembolic pulmonary hypertension (CTEPH) and should be performed in all patients undergoing PAH evaluation.[17] Although computed tomography pulmonary angiography (CTPA) is a useful test for acute pulmonary embolism, it is insensitive for the diagnosis of CTEPH. In a large retrospective study, ventilation perfusion scanning had a sensitivity and specificity for CTEPH of 96% compared

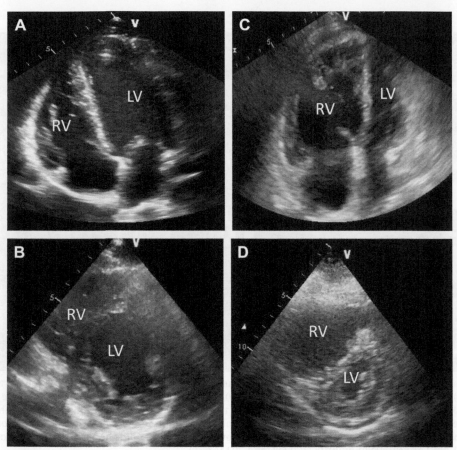

Fig. 3. Echocardiogram in a patient with PAH. (*A*) Apical four-chamber echocardiographic view of a normal heart demonstrating a normal-sized right ventricle (RV) and left ventricle (LV). (*B*) Short-axis echocardiographic image of a normal heart demonstrating a rounded LV and normal-appearing RV. (*C*) Apical four-chamber echocardiographic view from a patient with pulmonary hypertension demonstrating a markedly enlarged RV with a small, compressed LV. There is also enlargement of the right atrium. (*D*) Short-axis echocardiographic image from a patient with pulmonary hypertension demonstrating flattening of the interventricular septum and a D-shaped LV during systole and a large RV. (*From* Barnett CF, De Marco T. Pulmonary hypertension due to lung disease. In: Broaddus VC, Mason RJ, Ernst JD, et al, editors. Murray and Nadel's textbook of respiratory medicine. 6th edition. Philadelphia: W.B. Saunders; 2016. p. e1055; with permission.)

with 51% and 99%, respectively, for CTPA.[18] Reduced specificity of CTPA has also been described with false-positive findings in cases of pulmonary artery sarcoma and in PAH patients with proximal lining thrombus wrongly interpreted as evidence of CTEPH.[17] It is important to not miss a diagnosis of CTEPH, because without surgical pulmonary endarterectomy, CTEPH is a rapidly fatal disease.

Computed Tomography

Pulmonary artery dilation and cardiac chamber enlargement are common findings on chest CT in patients with PAH.[19] Findings of centrilobular ground glass opacities, interlobular septal thickening, and mediastinal adenopathy are suggestive of pulmonary veno-occlusive disease.

Abnormalities of the lung parenchyma or lymphadenopathy suggest an alternate etiology of PH such as parenchymal lung disease or sarcoidosis.

Cardiac Magnetic Resonance

Cardiac MRI has the advantage over echocardiography that it is not limited by acoustic widows. Although not available in many centers, cardiac MRI allows accurate and reproducible quantitative assessment of cardiac chambers, RV function, and identifying congenital structural heart disease (**Fig. 5**).[20]

TREATMENT

Treatment of patients with PAH requires that providers have specialized knowledge and

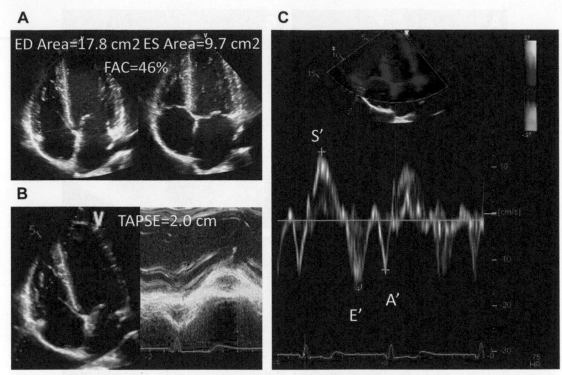

Fig. 4. Echocardiographic approaches to evaluating RV function. Examples of how to measure the fractional area change (*A*), tricuspid annular plane systolic excursion (*B*), and velocity of the tricuspid annular plane (*C*). (*Data from* Rudski LG, Lai WW, Afilalo J, et al. Guidelines for the echocardiographic assessment of the right heart in adults: a report from the American Society of Echocardiography endorsed by the European Association of Echocardiography, a registered branch of the European Society of Cardiology, and the Canadian Society of Echocardiography. J Am Soc Echocardiogr 2010;23(7):696 and 703.)

experience and access to the specialized resources, staff, and time necessary to adequately treat and follow up with these patients long term. Collaboration with a PH expert center is recommended for providers who do not have these resources.

Choice of treatment must take into consideration the underlying cause of PAH, comorbid illnesses, and concomitant medications. Careful review of the comprehensive diagnostic evaluation to identify and aggressively treat any comorbid conditions that may increase PAP is critical.

Recommendations for initial therapy depend on disease severity. The presence of high-risk features identifies patients in whom initial therapy with intravenous prostanoids or upfront combination therapy is recommended. High-risk features include:

- Syncope
- NYHA/World Health Organization (WHO) class IV
- Cardiopulmonary exercise testing with peak V_{O_2} less than 12 mL/kg/min
- Pericardial effusion
- TAPSE less than 15 mm
- RAP greater than 15 mm Hg
- Cardiac index ≤2 L/min/m2
- RV ejection fraction less than 35%

Table 3
Drugs used for vasodilator studies

Drug	Typical Dose	Adverse Effects
Inhaled NO	20 PPM for 5 min	Elevated left heart filling pressures
Intravenous epoprostenol	2–10 ng/kg/min	Hypotension, headache, flushing, nausea, lightheadedness
Intravenous adenosine	50–250 µg/kg/min	Chest tightness, dyspnea, atrioventricular block, hypotension

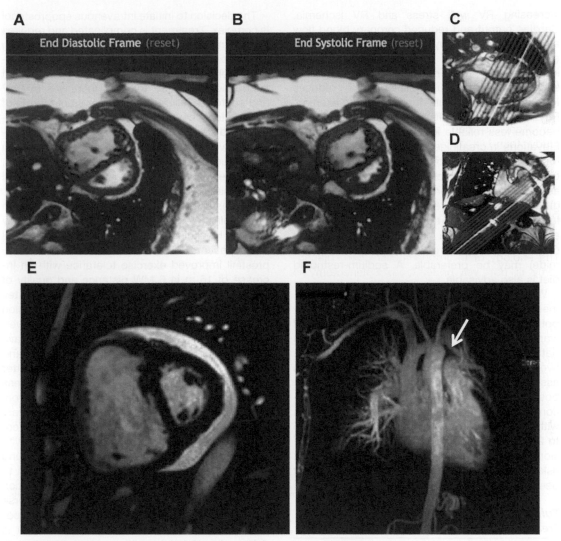

Fig. 5. Cardiac MRI in a patient with PAH. Quantification of RV end-diastolic (*A*) and end-systolic (*B*) volumes and reference planes (*C, D*). In this case, RV EDV and ESV measured in multiple planes were 316 mL and 207 mL, respectively, corresponding to a severely enlarged RV and an RV ejection fraction 34%. A large pericardial effusion in a patient with PAH (*E*). Diagnosis of partial anomalous pulmonary venous return (*white arrow*) causing PAH (*F*). EDV, end diastolic volume; ESV, end systolic volume.

After initiation of therapy, close and frequent follow-up is necessary. Many centers regularly assess exercise tolerance with frequent 6-minute walk tests (6 MW) and frequent echocardiography. Because PAH is a progressive disease, many patients will require intensification of treatment over time and should be cautioned to self-monitor and immediately report worsening symptoms. Treatment should be intensified until the following goals are met:

- NYHA/WHO class I or II
- Normal RV size and function
- 6 MW distance greater than 380 m to 400 m
- RAP less than 8 mm Hg
- CI greater than 2.5 to 3.0 L/min/m2

- Cardiopulmonary exercise testing with peak Vo_2 greater than 15 mL/min/kg and Ventilatory equivalent for carbon dioxide (VE/VCO_2) less than 45 L/min
- Brain natriuretic peptide normal

General Measures

Supplemental oxygen should be administered to maintain oxygen saturation greater than 92%. Oxygen may be required with sleep, exercise, or travel by air or to high altitude even in patients with normal resting saturation.

Diuretic treatment to optimize RV volumes and preload is important in all patients with PAH. Volume overload causes RV dilation leading to increasing RV wall stress and RV ischemia. Cardiac output and reduced coronary blood flow are further impaired by left heart underfilling secondary to pericardial constraint and ventricular interdependence.[21] Tricuspid regurgitation caused by tricuspid annular dilation further reduces forward cardiac output especially during exertion. Physical examination findings for volume overload become less reliable in advanced heart disease. Elevations in creatinine and hypotension that can result from fluid removal may further contribute to uncertainty about volume status so that invasive assessment of filling pressures may be required to guide therapy.[22] Unpredictable absorption of oral furosemide may limit the efficacy, in which case, addition of a thiazide diuretic or treatment with more potent loop diuretics (bumetanide or torsemide) may be preferable. A sodium-restricted diet is also advisable.

Warfarin treatment in PAH has been recommended based on postmortem findings of thrombotic vascular lesions. No randomized trials of warfarin in PAH have been performed, and clinical data comes largely from single-center retrospective studies. Recent data suggest that warfarin is associated with worse outcomes in SSc-PAH, possibly from increased bleeding complications.[23] Current guidelines recommend warfarin with a target international normalized ratio of 1.5 to 2.5 for patients with PAH; however, the decision must be individualized and take into account risk of bleeding. Novel anticoagulants have not been studied in PAH.

Pulmonary Arterial Hypertension Specific Treatments

Calcium channel blockers
High-dose calcium channel blockers are a useful treatment in some patients with IPAH and with a reduction in mPAP by at least 10 mm Hg to less than 40 mm Hg without a reduction in CO or increase PAWP during a vasodilator study. Calcium channel blockers should not be used to treat PAH that is not idiopathic in etiology because of lack of benefit in such patients.[24]

Prostacyclin pathway
Prostacyclin analogues Endogenous prostacyclin is synthesized by vascular endothelial cells and binds the prostacyclin receptor causing pulmonary artery vasodilation and inhibition of vascular smooth muscle cell proliferation. Epoprostenol improved survival compared with standard treatment in the landmark randomized 12-week trial of 81 patients.[25] These striking results established intravenous epoprostenol as the gold standard treatment of PAH.

The decision to initiate intravenous epoprostenol is complex. Treatment is complicated and requires a permanent central venous catheter, as the drug needs to be given via continuous infusion. Epoprostenol has a half-life of about 4 minutes, and interruption can lead to rapid increases in PAP and acute RV failure. Newer heat stable forms of epoprostenol have obviated the needs for refrigeration and ice packs, which were previously necessary. Adverse effects of prostainoids are common and include flushing, headache, jaw pain, diarrhea, and bone and joint pain but can often be managed with behavior modification and medications.

Treprostinil is a prostacyclin analogue that can be administered intravenously, subcutaneously (SC), by inhalation, or orally. In a randomized trial of 470 patients, 12 weeks of treatment with SC treprostinil improved exercise tolerance with an increase of 16 m in 6 MW distance and quality of life.[26] Administration via SC infusion eliminates the need for a central venous catheter. Infusion site pain may be challenging to manage; however, useful algorithms for site pain management have been developed.[27] Treprostinil is heat stable and has a half-life of 4.5 hours so may be a better choice for patients who do not have rapid access to medical care in the case of infusion interruption.

Inhaled treprostinil is delivered via a proprietary inhaler 4 to 6 times daily. In a randomized, placebo-controlled study of 235 patients with PAH, inhaled treprostinil in addition to background therapy with bosentan or sildenafil was found to improve exercise tolerance.[28] With the exception of cough caused by inhaled treprostinil, adverse effects of treprostinil are similar to those of epoprostenol. Iloprost is another prostanoid that is delivered by inhalation. In a placebo-controlled, randomized study, the 6 MW distance for PAH patients was 36.4 m further in iloprost-treated patients. However, in contrast to the study of inhaled treprostinil, no patients in the iloprost trial were on background PAH therapy likely causing the observed greater treatment effect compared with inhaled treprostinil. Because of a shorter half-life, iloprost must be administered 9 times daily, and use of the inhaler device is technically challenging, limiting the utility of this treatment.

The only oral prostanoid currently available in the United States is oral treprostinil. When studied in 349 treatment-naïve patients, treatment with oral treprostinil was associated with a 23 m improvement in 6 MW distance[29]; however, no improvements were found in 2 other studies of patients on background PAH therapy.[30,31] Study drop-out related to drug intolerance was common, and it has been proposed that lower starting doses could be associated with improved tolerance and treatment benefits, but this is supported by limited evidence.

Prostacyclin receptor agonist Selexipag is the first drug in a new class of oral prostacyclin receptor agonists. The results of a large 1156-person randomized, placebo-controlled trial showed a 40% reduction in the occurrence of a combined primary endpoint of clinical worsening or death in the treatment group.[32]

Endothelin receptor antagonists Endothelin receptor antagonists (ERA) block activity of the potent vasoconstrictor and mitogen endothelin. Bosentan, the first available oral therapy for PAH, was studied as monotherapy in the BREATHE-1 randomized, placebo-controlled trial of 213 treatment-naïve PAH patients. Compared with placebo, bosentan-treated patients walked 44 m further in 6 minutes, had improved functional class, and increased time to clinical worsening.[33] Monthly assessment of liver function tests is mandatory during treatment, and bosentan may result in fluid retention that can be managed with loop diuretics.

Effect on exercise tolerance in the 12-week randomized trial of ambrisentan was a 51-m increase in 6 MW distance for the 10 mg ambrisentan arm compared with placebo.[34] Ambrisentan is taken once daily and does not require liver function test monitoring.

The most recently approved ERA, macitentan, was studied in a large event-driven trial with a combined endpoint that included mortality. The event rate in the macitentan 10-mg group was 31.4% versus 46.4% in the placebo group with hospitalization accounting for most of these events. Patients in the macitentan 10 mg group also had a 22-m increase in 6 MW compared with placebo.[35] In contrast to bosentan, macitentan does not affect liver function results, and is less likely to cause fluid retention compared with bosentan and ambrisentan.

Because of severe teratogenicity, prescribers of ERAs must ensure patients use adequate contraception and monitor for pregnancy during treatment.

Nitric oxide pathway Nitric oxide (NO), synthesized by pulmonary vascular endothelial cells, activates soluble guanylate cyclase (sGC) to produce 3'5'-cyclic guanosine monophosphate, which inhibits vasoconstriction, cellular proliferation, and migration. Complex delivery systems and the short half-life of inhaled NO make it impractical for the treatment of ambulatory patients; however, NO effects may be augmented by blocking the breakdown of 3'5'-cyclic guanosine monophosphate by phosphodiesterase type 5 inhibition (PDE-5) or direct activation of sGC.

Phosphodiesterase inhibitors Sildenafil was the second oral medication approved for the treatment of PAH after a randomized, controlled trial of 278 patients that found a 45-m improvement in 6 MW distance compared with placebo.[36] Although the US Food and Drug Administration–approved dose of sildenafil is 20 mg 3 times daily, it has been used in higher doses, which is thought by some experts to confer additional clinical benefits (**Table 4**). Tadalafil was studied in a 405-patient, 16-week randomized, controlled trial that found a similar 33-m improvement in 6 MW compared with placebo.[37] Both medications are well tolerated with major side effects of headache and nasal congestion. Advantages to tadalafil are that it can be administered once daily compared with 3 times a day for sildenafil and has fewer drug interactions with protease inhibitors used to treat HIV.

Guanylate cyclase agonists Riociguat directly activates soluble guanylate cyclase so may have improved efficacy in NO-deficient states such as endothelial dysfunction associated with PH. In a randomized trial of 443 patients, riociguat added to background therapy improved 6 MW by 30 m compared with placebo. Riociguat was frequently stopped for hypotension, so starting at a low dose with slow titration every 2 weeks is recommended. Riociguat cannot be used in combination with PDE-5 inhibitors because of the risk of severe hypotension. Riociguat is also teratogenic, and prescribers must ensure required contraception is used and patients are monitored for pregnancy during treatment.[38]

Combination therapy Response to PAH monotherapy is often unsatisfactory, and management with addition of drug from other therapeutic classes is recommended.[39] The AMBITION study evaluated up-front combination therapy with ambriesentan and tadalafil versus monotherapy in treatment-naïve patients. The clinical trial found that up-front combination treatment strategy approach reduced death and clinical worsening events by 50% and improve exercise tolerance compared with initial monotherapy. Data from a small single-center trial also recently showed 100% 3-year survival in 18 patients with advanced PAH treated with up-front triple combination consisting of intravenous epoprostenol, sildenafil, and bosentan.[40] These data suggest that up-front combination therapy with tadalafil and ambrisentan should be considered for most patients, and triple therapy is reasonable in carefully selected patients.

Table 4
US Food and Drug Administration–approved drugs for the treatment of pulmonary arterial hypertension

Drug Trial Name (N)	Trial Outcomes	Clinical Pearls
Endothelin receptor antagonists		
Bosentan BREATHE-1 (213)	Improved 6 MW distance Improved dyspnea Delayed clinical worsening	Hepatic toxicity Teratogenic Fluid retention, peripheral edema, anemia, nasal congestion, sinusitis, flushing Monthly transaminase monitoring required
Ambrisentan ARIES-1 (202) ARIES-2 (192)	Improved 6 MW walk distance Delayed clinical worsening Improved hemodynamics No effect on transaminases	Teratogenic Fluid retention, peripheral edema, anemia, nasal congestion, sinusitis, flushing
Macitentan SERAPHIN (742)	Reduced incidence of composite endpoint of death, atrial septostomy, lung transplantation, intravenous or SQ prostanoid therapy or worsening PAH	Teratogenic Headache, nasopharyngitis, anemia
Phosphodiesterase-5 inhibitors		
Sildenafil SUPER-1 (278)	Improved 6 MW walk distance Improved dyspnea Improved hemodynamics	No delay in clinical worsening end point Headache, flushing, dyspepsia, epistaxis, visual disturbance Interactions with protease inhibitors
Tadalafil PHIRST (405)	Improved 6 MW distance Improved time to clinical worsening Improved hemodynamics Improved quality of life	Headache, myalgias, flushing, dyspepsia, epistaxis, visual disturbance

Soluble guanylate cyclase agonists

Drug (Trial)	Efficacy	Adverse effects / Notes
Riociguat PATENT-1 and 2 (443)	Improved 6 MW distance Improved hemodynamics Improved time to clinical worsening Improved quality of life Reduced brain natriuretic peptide Improved WHO class Improved dyspnea	Teratogenic Headache, dyspepsia, edema, dyspepsia, nausea, dizziness Severe hypotension with PDE-5 inhibitors

Prostanoids

Drug (Trial)	Efficacy	Adverse effects / Notes
Epoprostenol, intravenous (81)	Improved 6 MW distance Improved dyspnea Improved hemodynamics Improved survival	Indwelling central line Pump malfunction Flushing, jaw pain, thrombocytopenia, headache, dizziness, nausea/vomiting/diarrhea, abdominal pain, hypotension, rash
Treprostinil, intravenous or subcutaneous (70)	Improved 6 MW distance Improved dyspnea Improved hemodynamics	Indwelling central line or subcutaneous catheter Pain, erythema at infusion site (subcutaneous) Flushing, jaw pain, thrombocytopenia headache, dizziness, nausea/vomiting/diarrhea, abdominal pain, hypotension, rash
Treprostinil, inhaled Triumph (470)	Improved 6 MW distance Improved quality of life Administration 4 times daily	No delay in clinical worsening or dyspnea No change in functional class Cough, headache, nausea, dizziness, flushing, throat irritation or pain
Treprostinil, oral FREEDOM-M (349)	Improved 6 MW distance	No additional benefits when added to PDE-5 or ERA Headache, nausea, diarrhea, jaw pain
Iloprost, inhaled (203)	Improved composite endpoint of 6 MW distance and dyspnea	Administration 6–9 times daily Cough, headache, nausea, dizziness, flushing, throat irritation or pain

IP Prostacyclin receptor agonist

Drug (Trial)	Efficacy	Adverse effects / Notes
Selexipag GRIPHON (1156)	Reduced incidence of composite endpoint of any complication of PAH or death	Headache, diarrhea, nausea, jaw pain.

SUMMARY

Modern therapies permit improved long-term survival in patients with PAH. Key to optimizing outcomes in patients with PAH is early diagnosis and early and aggressive PAH treatment provided in collaboration with a PAH care center treatment.

SUPPLEMENTARY DATA

Supplementary data related to this article can be found at http://dx.doi.org/10.1016/j.ccl.2016.04.006.

REFERENCES

1. Deaño RC, Glassner-Kolmin C, Rubenfire M, et al. Referral of patients with pulmonary hypertension diagnoses to tertiary pulmonary hypertension centers: the multicenter repherral study. JAMA Intern Med 2013;173:887–93.
2. McLaughlin VV, Langer A, Tan M, et al. Contemporary trends in the diagnosis and management of pulmonary arterial hypertension: an initiative to close the care gap. Chest 2013;143:324–32.
3. Hoeper MM, Bogaard HJ, Condliffe R, et al. Definitions and diagnosis of pulmonary hypertension. J Am Coll Cardiol 2013;62:D42–50.
4. Coghlan JG, Denton CP, Grünig E, et al. Evidence-based detection of pulmonary arterial hypertension in systemic sclerosis: the DETECT study. Ann Rheum Dis 2014;73(7):1340–9.
5. Lau EMT, Humbert M, Celermajer DS. Early detection of pulmonary arterial hypertension. Nat Rev Cardiol 2015;12:143–55.
6. McLaughlin VV, Archer SL, Badesch DB, et al. ACCF/AHA 2009 expert consensus document on pulmonary hypertension: a report of the American College of Cardiology Foundation Task Force on Expert Consensus Documents and the American Heart Association: developed in collaboration with the American College of Chest Physicians, American Thoracic Society, Inc., and the Pulmonary Hypertension Association. Circulation 2009;119: 2250–94.
7. McLaughlin VV, Shah SJ, Souza R, et al. Management of pulmonary arterial hypertension. J Am Coll Cardiol 2015;65:1976–97.
8. Fisher MR, Forfia PR, Chamera E, et al. Accuracy of Doppler echocardiography in the hemodynamic assessment of pulmonary hypertension. Am J Respir Crit Care Med 2009;179:615–21.
9. Rudski LG, Lai WW, Afilalo J, et al. Guidelines for the echocardiographic assessment of the right heart in adults: a report from the American Society of Echocardiography: endorsed by the European Association of Echocardiography, a registered branch of the European Society of Cardiology, and the Canadian Society of Echocardiography. J Am Soc Echocardiogr 2010;23:685–713.
10. Lam CSP, Roger VL, Rodeheffer RJ, et al. Pulmonary hypertension in heart failure with preserved ejection fraction: a community-based study. J Am Coll Cardiol 2009;53:1119–26.
11. Jacobs W, Konings TC, Heymans MW, et al. Noninvasive identification of left-sided heart failure in a population suspected of pulmonary arterial hypertension. Eur Respir J 2015;46:422–30.
12. Hoeper MM, Lee SH, Voswinckel R, et al. Complications of right heart catheterization procedures in patients with pulmonary hypertension in experienced centers. J Am Coll Cardiol 2006;48:2546–52.
13. Hoeper MM, Maier R, Tongers J, et al. Determination of cardiac output by the fick method, thermodilution, and acetylene rebreathing in pulmonary hypertension. Am J Respir Crit Care Med 1999; 160:535–41.
14. Ryan JJ, Rich JD, Thiruvoipati T, et al. Current practice for determining pulmonary capillary wedge pressure predisposes to serious errors in the classification of patients with pulmonary hypertension. Am Heart J 2012;163:589–94.
15. Sun X-G, Hansen JE, Oudiz RJ, et al. Pulmonary function in primary pulmonary hypertension. J Am Coll Cardiol 2003;41:1028–35.
16. Atwood JCW, McCrory D, Garcia JGN, et al. Pulmonary artery hypertension and sleep-disordered breathing: ACCP evidence-based clinical practice guidelines. Chest 2004;126:72S–7S.
17. Kim NH, Delcroix M, Jenkins DP, et al. Chronic thromboembolic pulmonary hypertension. J Am Coll Cardiol 2013;62(25 Suppl):D92–9.
18. Tunariu N, Gibbs SJR, Win Z, et al. Ventilation–perfusion scintigraphy is more sensitive than multidetector CTPA in detecting chronic thromboembolic pulmonary disease as a treatable cause of pulmonary hypertension. J Nucl Med 2007;48:680–4.
19. Rajaram S, Swift AJ, Condliffe R, et al. CT features of pulmonary arterial hypertension and its major subtypes: a systematic CT evaluation of 292 patients from the ASPIRE Registry. Thorax 2014; 70(4):382–7.
20. Vonk-Noordegraaf A, Souza R. Cardiac magnetic resonance imaging: what can it add to our knowledge of the right ventricle in pulmonary arterial hypertension? Am J Cardiol 2012;110:25S–31S.
21. Andersen MJ, Nishimura RA, Borlaug BA. The hemodynamic basis of exercise intolerance in tricuspid regurgitation. Circ Heart Fail 2014;7:911–7.
22. Haddad F, Doyle R, Murphy DJ, et al. Right ventricular function in cardiovascular disease, Part II: pathophysiology, clinical importance, and management of right ventricular failure. Circulation 2008;117: 1717–31.

23. Roldan T, Landzberg MJ, Deicicchi DJ, et al. Anticoagulation in patients with pulmonary arterial hypertension: an update on current knowledge. J Heart Lung Transplant 2016;35(2):151–64.

24. Montani D, Savale L, Natali D, et al. Long-term response to calcium-channel blockers in non-idiopathic pulmonary arterial hypertension. Eur Heart J 2010;31:1898–907.

25. Barst RJ, Rubin LJ, Long WA, et al. A comparison of continuous intravenous epoprostenol (prostacyclin) with conventional therapy for primary pulmonary hypertension. N Engl J Med 1996;334:296–301.

26. Simonneau G, Barst RJ, Galie N, et al. Continuous subcutaneous infusion of treprostinil, a prostacyclin analogue, in patients with pulmonary arterial hypertension. Am J Respir Crit Care Med 2002;165:800–4.

27. White RJ, Levin Y, Wessman K, et al. Subcutaneous treprostinil is well tolerated with infrequent site changes and analgesics. Pulm Circ 2013;3:611–21.

28. McLaughlin VV, Benza RL, Rubin LJ, et al. Addition of Inhaled treprostinil to oral therapy for pulmonary arterial hypertension: a randomized controlled clinical trial. J Am Coll Cardiol 2010;55:1915–22.

29. Jing Z-C, Parikh K, Pulido T, et al. Efficacy and safety of oral treprostinil monotherapy for the treatment of pulmonary arterial hypertension: a randomized, controlled trial. Circulation 2013;127:624–33.

30. Tapson VF, Jing Z-C, Xu K-F, et al. Oral treprostinil for the treatment of pulmonary arterial hypertension in patients receiving background endothelin receptor antagonist and phosphodiesterase type 5 inhibitor therapy (the freedom-c2 study): a randomized controlled trial. Chest 2013;144:952–8.

31. Tapson VF, Torres F, Kermeen F, et al. Oral treprostinil for the treatment of pulmonary arterial hypertension in patients on background endothelin receptor antagonist and/or phosphodiesterase type 5 inhibitor therapy (the freedom-c study): a randomized controlled trial. Chest 2012;142:1383–90.

32. Sitbon O, Channick R, Chin KM, et al. Selexipag for the treatment of pulmonary arterial hypertension. N Engl J Med 2015;373:2522–33.

33. Rubin LJ, Badesch DB, Barst RJ, et al. Bosentan therapy for pulmonary arterial hypertension. N Engl J Med 2002;346:896–903.

34. Galiè N, Olschewski H, Oudiz RJ, et al. Ambrisentan for the treatment of pulmonary arterial hypertension: results of the ambrisentan in pulmonary arterial hypertension, randomized, double-blind, placebo-controlled, multicenter, efficacy (ARIES) study 1 and 2. Circulation 2008;117:3010–9.

35. Pulido T, Adzerikho I, Channick RN, et al. Macitentan and morbidity and mortality in pulmonary arterial hypertension. N Engl J Med 2013;369:809–18.

36. Galie N, Ghofrani HA, Torbicki A, et al. Sildenafil citrate therapy for pulmonary arterial hypertension. N Engl J Med 2005;353:2148–57.

37. Galiè N, Brundage BH, Ghofrani HA, et al. Tadalafil therapy for pulmonary arterial hypertension. Circulation 2009;119:2894–903.

38. Ghofrani H-A, Galiè N, Grimminger F, et al. Riociguat for the treatment of pulmonary arterial hypertension. N Engl J Med 2013;369:330–40.

39. Ghofrani H-A, Humbert M. The role of combination therapy in managing pulmonary arterial hypertension. Eur Respir Rev 2014;23:469–75.

40. Sitbon O, Jaïs X, Savale L, et al. Upfront triple combination therapy in pulmonary arterial hypertension: a pilot study. Eur Respir J 2014;43:1691–7.

Pulmonary Hypertension and Congenital Heart Disease

Todd S. Roth, MD[a],*, Jamil A. Aboulhosn, MD[b]

KEYWORDS

- Adults with congenital heart disease (ACHD)
- Pulmonary arterial hypertension (PAH)
- Eisenmenger syndrome (ES)
- Targeted, catheter-based, surgical therapies

KEY POINTS

- Updates in definition and classification.
- Pathophysiologic and anatomic considerations.
- Medical treatment.
- Catheter-based and surgical-based strategies.

INTRODUCTION

The population growth of adults with congenital heart disease (ACHD) continues to accelerate, unveiling a group of patients with unique and complex medical problems. On its current trajectory, the ACHD population is accelerating at an approximate rate of 5% per year.[1] More than 1 million adults in the United States now have congenital heart defects with an estimated 10% having pulmonary arterial hypertension (PAH) and as many as 30% of unrepaired patients having PAH.[2–4] Of this subset of patients, nearly 50% will progress to Eisenmenger syndrome (ES), a condition resulting in right to left shunting, profound cyanosis, and clinical deterioration.[5] It is paramount to identify and optimally treat these patients so as to improve quality of life and reduce morbidity and mortality.

The goal of this article was to provide a current overview of PAH associated with CHD (PAH-CHD). An updated definition and classification of pulmonary hypertension (PH)/PAH is discussed along with a brief review of essential pathophysiologic and anatomic points. Additionally, relevant diagnostic and management considerations are examined.

UPDATED DEFINITIONS AND CLASSIFICATION

The most recent world meeting on PH was held in 2013 at the 5th World Symposium on Pulmonary Hypertension (5WSPH) in Nice, France. In part, to address the physiologic impact pulmonary vascular resistance (PVR) has on the management of patients with PAH-CHD, it was recommended to include the hemodynamic criterion for the subset of patients with PH having PAH with the following hemodynamic profile[6]:

- Mean pulmonary arterial pressure (PAP) ≥25 mm Hg
- Left ventricular end-diastolic pressure or pulmonary capillary wedge pressure ≤15 mm Hg
- Elevated PVR (PVR >3 Wood units [WU])

The subgroup of CHD encompassing left-sided obstructive lesions such as Shone complex

[a] Memorial Cardiac and Vascular Institute, Joe DiMaggio Children's Hospital Adult Congenital Heart Disease Center, 3501 Johnson Street, Hollywood, FL 33021, USA; [b] Ahmanson/UCLA Adult Congenital Heart Disease Center, Medicine and Pediatrics David Geffen School of Medicine at UCLA, 100 UCLA Medical Plaza, Suite 630, Los Angeles, CA 90095, USA
* Corresponding author. Memorial Cardiac and Vascular Institute, Joe DiMaggio Children's Hospital Adult Congenital Heart Disease Center, 3501 Johnson Street, Hollywood, FL 33021.
E-mail address: troth@mhs.net

Cardiol Clin 34 (2016) 391–400
http://dx.doi.org/10.1016/j.ccl.2016.04.002

(the combined presence of parachute mitral valve, supravalvular mitral ring, subaortic stenosis, and coarctation of the aorta) was reclassified from group 1 (PAH) to Group 2 (PH due to left heart disease).[7]

Additionally at the 5WSPH, an updated clinical subclassification of PAH-CHD was proposed to better delineate the 4 phenotypes (**Box 1**).[7]

ANATOMIC AND PATHOPHYSIOLOGIC FEATURES

The anatomic defects in CHD, whether associated with PH or not, can vary quite broadly. It is important to understand the circulatory principles that predispose patients with CHD to PAH, as this allows for improved fundamental knowledge of the concomitant anatomic lesions and appropriate management thereof.

Most commonly, PAH-CHD results from uncorrected, large systemic-to-pulmonary shunts (LSPS) either at the ventricular or great arterial level (**Figs. 1** and **2**).[8,9] In this physiologic

---

> **Box 1**
> **Clinical classification of congenital systemic-to-pulmonary shunts associated with pulmonary arterial hypertension**
>
> *Postoperative*
> - Congenital heart disease is repaired
> - Pulmonary arterial hypertension (PAH) persists after surgery
> - PAH recurs/develops months or years after surgery
>
> *Coincidental*
> - Marked pulmonary vascular resistance (PVR) increase in the presence of a small cardiac defect
> - The defect does not account for the elevated PVR
>
> *Left-to-right shunts*
> - Moderate-to-large defects
> - Mild to moderately increased PVR
> - Cyanosis is not a feature
>
> *Eisenmenger syndrome*
> - All large intracardiac and extracardiac defects
> - Reversal or bidirectional shunting
> - Secondary erythrocytosis
>
> *Data from* Simonneau G, Gatzoulis MA, Adatia I. Updated clinical classification of pulmonary hypertension. J Am Coll Cardiol 2013;62(25 Suppl):D34–41.

---

arrangement, there is an increase in pulmonary blood flow at systemic-level pressure with subsequent proliferative changes in the pulmonary architecture leading to severe increases in PVR and often resulting in reversal of shunt direction (ES).[10,11] An estimated 48% of patients with large unrepaired ventricular septal defects and PH will go on to develop ES.[8] In 1958, Paul Wood[11] more specifically described ES as PH with PAP at systemic levels attributable to PVR greater than 10 WU and consequently reversed or bidirectional shunting at the ventricular or great arterial level, collectively referred to as "central shunts." Professor Wood[11] took great pains to distinguish the pathophysiology and natural history of "low-pressure" atrial level shunts from central shunts; the former not commonly associated with severe PAH or cyanosis, whereas the latter are almost always associated with PAH and cyanosis if not repaired early in life.

There is increasing support for the concept that pressure rather than flow is the more important etiologic factor in developing PAH-CHD. A growing body of evidence has shown that endothelin-1 (ET-1) production is increased in patients with PH, increased PVR, and ES.[17,18] More recently, Fratz and colleagues[19] showed that mean PAP had the greatest effect on ET-1 concentrations with flow having no effect on ET-1 production in 56 patients with CHD and normal PVR.

In contrast to LSPS, pre-tricuspid valve defects (see **Fig. 1**), are typically low-pressure lesions, less likely to result in PAH. When these lesions advance to PAH, it occurs at a later age.[20] Data from the CONCOR registry on Dutch ACHDs showed a 7% risk for developing PAH with an associated atrial septal defect (ASD), an 11% risk with a ventricular septal defect (VSD), and a 41% risk with an atrioventricular septal defect (AVSD). Furthermore, those with a VSD are more than 2 times as likely to develop ES than with an ASD.[8] Despite this statistical relationship, those patients with pre–tricuspid valve lesions that develop ES appear to have worse outcomes. In the Spanish Registry of Pulmonary Arterial Hypertension (REHAP) (240 patients across 31 hospitals in Spain), Alonso-Gonzalez and colleagues[21] demonstrated a 2.6-fold higher mortality for patients with pre–tricuspid valve lesions compared with those with post–tricuspid valve shunts.

These findings have been reproduced[11,20,22,23] and necessitate brief discussion. Paul Wood[11] in 1958 offered an explanation why patients with pre–tricuspid valve lesions were less likely to develop PAH, and when PAH does occur, why it occurs at a later age than in patients with post–tricuspid valve lesions. In the patients with PAH,

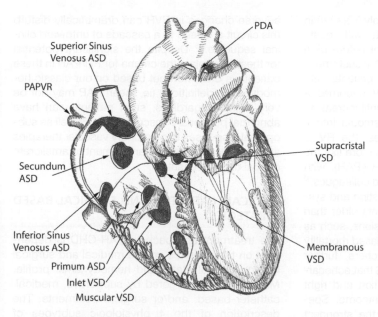

Fig. 1. VSD, ASD, and PDA. VSDs are the most common defects (42%), among patients with PAH and septal defects.[8] Large VSDs, in combination with other complex anatomies (double-outlet RV, truncus arteriosus, AVSDs, d-TGA/VSD, or single ventricles) that are associated with unobstructed pulmonary blood flow, behave in the same physiologic manner as large isolated or multiple VSDs. PDA accounts for 5% to 10%.[8] If unguarded, the cascade of pulmonary vascular disease unfolds, leading to a 20% risk of PAH and ES.[12] Aortopulmonary window is rare with high risk to develop pulmonary vascular disease if left uncorrected.[13] Five anatomic subtypes of ASDs exist; secundum ASD accounts for 75% of defects. Ostium primum defects, often accompanied by AVSDs, occur in 20% of cases. Sinus venosus defects (usually superior) occur in 5% of patients and of interest, have been shown to have the highest risk of the ASD family in developing PAH.[14] The most rare type is the coronary sinus ASD. Partial anomalous pulmonary venous return is a rare lesion, 0.6% to 0.8%[15] with multiple variations. Anomalous veins may drain into the right atrium, left innominate vein, coronary sinus, superior vena cava, or the inferior vena cava (Scimitar syndrome).

he surmised that diastolic right ventricular compliance is abnormal as a result of slow right ventricular remodeling in the newborn. Because shunt volume at the atrial level is driven in part by the relative compliance of the right and left ventricles, poor right ventricular compliance is associated with decreased left-to-right shunting. This absence of high pressure and high flow in the pulmonary arterial circuit of the newborn allows the PVR to fall as the pulmonary arterial vasculature remodels to a low resistance circuit. With time, the right ventricular compliance improves and pulmonary blood flow increases due to left-to-right shunting across the atrial septum. Increased pulmonary blood flow does not result in increased pulmonary arterial resistance for the first few decades, but eventually increases in PVR may occur.[11] Perhaps counterintuitive, this could help explain why patients with an

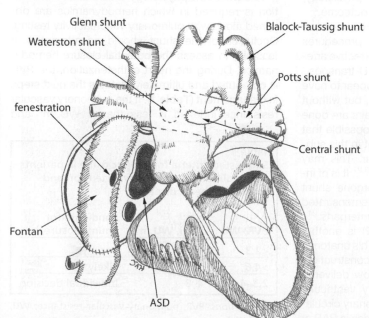

Fig. 2. Surgical shunts and Fontan anastomoses. Blalock-Taussig shunt (BTS), first performed in 1944, involved fashioning the right subclavian artery to the right pulmonary artery, later replaced by a synthetic conduit, termed the modified BTS.[16] This type of shunt allows for more restricted pulmonary flow and thus a lower risk profile to develop PAH. The Potts shunt: descending thoracic aorta to the left pulmonary artery. Cooley-Waterston shunt: communication between the posterior aspect of the ascending aorta and the right PA.[16] Central shunt: anastomosed the ascending aorta and the main PA.

ASD and severe PAH fare considerably worse than their VSD counterparts. In patients with post–tricuspid valve shunts, PH is present before birth and thus the right ventricle (RV) is "accustomed" to a high afterload, in contrast to patients with atrial-level shunts in whom the RV becomes a thin-walled volume pump at birth, until increasing PVR later in life challenges it to remodel into a high-pressure pump. In such cases, the RV is said to be poorly adapted, behaving more like the RV in a patient with idiopathic PAH (iPAH), with early dilation and failure.[21] Moceri and colleagues[20] demonstrated that significant RV dilation and systolic dysfunction can occur in patients older than 48 years with pre–tricuspid valve lesions, such as an ASD. This is associated with increased mortality in these patients. These researchers further demonstrated in 181 patients with ES that echocardiographic assessment of RV function and right heart chamber size can predict outcome. Specifically, a composite score using the strongest echocardiographic predictors; tricuspid annular plane systolic excursion less than 15 mm, ratio of RV systolic:diastolic duration ≥ 1.5, right atrium area ≥ 25 cm^2, and right atrium/left atrium ≥ 1.5, was shown to increase the risk of death by more than threefold.[24]

Other CHD subtypes associated with an increased risk for developing PAH include repaired cardiac defects and small, restrictive defects thought to be hemodynamically insignificant. These small defects are termed coincidental lesions. Nonetheless, both entities are prone to developing PAH. This type of PAH is often severe and can behave similarly to iPAH both in physiology, response to treatment, and long-term outcome.[25]

A particular group of patients with CHD who have undergone palliative atrial switch procedures (Mustard or Senning repairs) and/or corrective arterial switch operations in childhood for D-transposition of the great arteries group, also appear to have an increased risk for developing PAH, but without clear causation, as most of these repairs are done within the first few weeks of life. It is possible that pulmonary vascular disease is present in this subset of patients before surgical repair. This may occur in up to 10% of these patients.[26,27] It is of interest that patients who have undergone shunt closure and develop PAH-CHD have demonstrated worse survival rates than their ES counterparts.[21]

The Fontan circulation (see **Fig. 2**) is another important physiologic consideration. This anatomic arrangement, regardless of surgical construction, relies on passive systemic venous flow delivered at a low pressure (no subpulmonary ventricular pump) to adequately supply the pulmonary circulation. In these patients, marginal increases in PAP or adverse changes in PVR can dramatically disturb this circuit and lead to a cascade of untoward clinical sequelae.[28] Despite the significant potential for these sequelae, the criteria for PH/PAH in these patients is often not met based on our classic hemodynamic definitions (ie, mean PAP may not be very high). Regardless, such patients can have abnormal pulmonary vascular beds as well as suboptimal responses to pulmonary vascular therapies and require aggressive management to ameliorate clinical decompensation.

MEDICAL, CATHETER, AND SURGICAL-BASED STRATEGIES

The treatment approach to PAH-CHD is dependent on the patient's unique medical and surgical history, clinical state, and hemodynamic profile. Management is targeted by supportive, medical, catheter-based, and/or surgical treatments. The description of the 4 physiologic subtypes of PAH-CHD described previously in **Box 1** is a useful subclassification tool that helps clarify and inform the various management strategies appropriate to each physiologic condition.

In group A (PAH after corrective surgery) and group B (coincidental PAH with small defects), there is no indication for catheter-based or surgical procedures. Patients with these entities behave physiologically similar to iPAH and therefore the World Health Organization group 1 (PAH) treatment algorithm is followed.[29] Group C reflects PAH due to a left-to-right shunt from a moderate to large defect with sequelae of mild to moderately elevated PVR.

To confirm the physiology, a cardiac catheterization is required in which hemodynamics are obtained along with pulmonary vasoreactivity testing. Occlusion of the shunt should be attempted, if feasible, to assess the potential closure hemodynamics. During the heart catheterization, the PVR is computed and ultimately dictates the next steps in management (**Table 1**). If the pulmonary vascular resistance indexed is less than 4 WU m^2 and

Table 1
Suggested criteria for shunt closure in patients with pulmonary arterial hypertension and congenital heart disease

PVR, WU	PVRi, WU m^2	Candidate for Shunt Closure
<2.3	<4	Yes
>4.6	>8	Likely not
2.3–4.6	4–8	Individual decision

Abbreviations: PVR, pulmonary vascular resistance; WU, Wood unit.

surgery is chosen, specific issues in the ACHD population should be understood, especially in the presence of reoperation. Reentry into the chest is complicated by extensive scar tissue from prior surgeries as well as the development of extensive collaterization, which can lead to chest wall bleeding that is tedious to control. The proximity of the heart to the sternum is often problematic and requires meticulous attention and creative alternative approaches to avoid excessive bleeding and achieve control of the circulatory system. In addition, cardiopulmonary bypass times are significantly increased and the need for blood products is as well.[30] For these reasons, the option of catheter-based intervention (CBI) can be quite appealing and sometimes preferred if performed safely by an interventionalist with experience in CHD procedures.

The choice to proceed with CBI is supported by data showing these interventions yield shorter hospital stays, fewer procedural complications, and equivalent long-term outcomes compared with surgery.[14,15,31] The lesions typically amenable to CBI include secundum ASD, VSD, and patent

ductus arteriosus (PDA).[32] **Table 2** demonstrates the clinical and hemodynamic profiles that support intervention for each of these lesions.[33]

Of interest is the treatment decision for the patient with a moderately elevated PVRi between 4 to 8 WU m^2. This cohort is especially challenging given that results of interventions have been mixed, and those left with residual PAH after correction carry an extremely poor prognosis,[34–36] with even worse reported outcomes than if left uncorrected.[37] Additionally, medical treatment alone has not been well-studied in this subgroup.

Despite these limitations, the impressive advances in targeted therapies, albeit best studied in ES, makes a nonsurgical-interventional (catheter-based vs surgical) approach attractive. Currently, there is no clear consensus regarding when device closure of a defect becomes acceptable following medical treatment of PAH, although a large number of successful anecdotal experiences have been reported in the past decade,[38] leaving management institutionally biased. Of some help is a recent study by D'Alto and colleagues,[39] which showed that patients who developed PAH late after ASD or VSD closure had baseline PVR $\geq$ 5 WU, PVRi $\geq$6 WU m^2, and PVR:systemic vascular resistance (SVR) greater than 0.33.

Group D represents ES. Early attempts at surgical closure of these patients with ES with reversed shunts were met with an unacceptably high risk of mortality and the practice was quickly abandoned. Thereafter, the condition was deemed "irreversible," and even though this common wisdom is currently being challenged (as described previously), most of ES cases are deemed too high risk, and closure is contraindicated.[40,41] There are published case series describing successful partial closure with surgically placed fenestrated patches but this is not a widespread practice.

Therefore, this subgroup is most commonly treated with supportive care for their multisystem

Table 2
Indications for intervention in congenital shunt defects

Defect	Indications for Intervention
Secundum ASD	Qp:Qs $\geq$1.5:1.0 RVE, RAE Mild-moderate Pulmonary HTN: PAP <2/3 systemic pressure PVR <2/3 systemic Paradoxic embolism
Ventricular septal defect	Qp:Qs $\geq$1.5:1.0 LAE, LVE Mild-moderate pulmonary HTN: PAP <2/3 systemic PVR <2/3 systemic Paradoxic embolism DOE AR
Patent ductus arteriosus	Qp:Qs $\geq$1.5:1.0 LAE, LVE Mild-moderate pulmonary HTN: PAP <2/3 systemic PVR <2/3 systemic SVT/DOE

Abbreviations: AR, aortic regurgitation; DOE, dyspnea on exertion; HTN, hypertension; LAE, left atrial enlargement; LVE, left ventricular enlargement; PAP, pulmonary artery pressure; PDA, patent ductus arteriosus; PVR, pulmonary vascular resistance; Qp, pulmonary blood flow; Qs, systemic blood flow; RAE, right atrial enlargement; RVE, Right ventricular enlargement; SVT, supraventricular tachycardia.

Table 3
Supportive therapies for Eisenmenger therapy

Area of Concern	Therapy
Immunizations	Influenza, pneumococcal
Endocarditis	Provide prophylaxis
Hyperviscosity	Treat with symptoms
Iron deficiency	Iron supplementation
Physical activity	Symptom limited
Volume status	Avoid dehydration
Pregnancy	Contraindicated
Anticoagulation	Reserve treatment for other indications

comorbidities (**Table 3**) and otherwise focus is concentrated on targeted therapies.

There have been numerous studies looking at targeted therapies for group D patients. Several of these studies have demonstrated efficacy with phosphodiesterase type 5 inhibitors (PDE-5i), endothelin receptor antagonists (ERAs), and prostanoids in the treatment of ES. This includes the important findings of the BREATHE-5 trial, the first randomized, double-blind, placebo-controlled study in patients with ES where it was demonstrated that the endothelin antagonist bosentan significantly reduced PVR and improved exercise capacity at 16 weeks with extension of these benefits seen up to 1 year follow-up.[42] This work has helped formulate an evidence-based treatment approach in this challenging group (**Fig. 3**).

In recent years, additional contributions have added to the list of several important ongoing and completed trials to date (**Table 4**).

In those group D patients who fail treatment and continue to deteriorate, heart and heart-lung (block) transplantation become the final therapeutic options.[50] Patients with ES may be offered lung transplantation with repair of the cardiac defect or heart-lung transplantation. The success of either approach in these patients has been limited.[51]

Given the advancements in the management of PH and the limited success of these operations, mainly the sickest patients who fail to stabilize or improve on pulmonary arterial vascular therapy are considered for candidacy. Finally, the potential roles of ventricular assist devices and the total artificial heart in patients with CHD and PAH are still under investigation, with promising early results.[52,53]

With regard to the unique Fontan circuit (see **Fig. 2**), increases in PAP or PVR in can have deleterious effects that lead to Fontan failure, characterized by congestive heart failure, arrhythmias, ascites, protein-losing enteropathy, and death.[54] Although multiple nonrandomized studies have shown efficacy in exercise and functional capacity in this population,[55,56] 2 randomized trials (one evaluating bosentan, and the other sildenafil) have failed to demonstrate efficacy.[57,58] Despite these mixed results, a more recent and robust randomized, placebo-controlled, double-blind study, TEMPO (Treatment with Endothelin Receptor Antagonist in Fontan Patients), showed improved exercise capacity, exercise time, and functional class.[59] This study suggests that this challenging group of patients with PAH-CHD may indeed derive benefit from pulmonary vascular therapy.

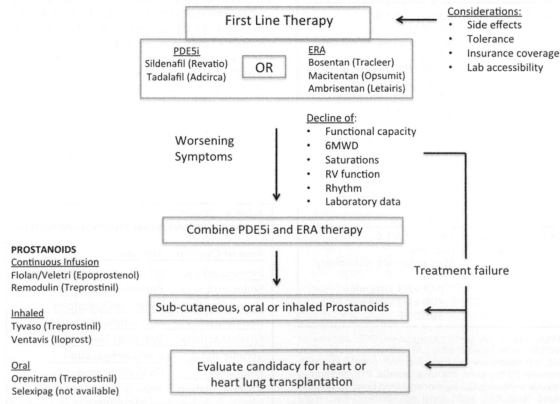

Fig. 3. Suggested treatment algorithm for PAH and ES. 6MWD, 6-minute walk distance.

Table 4
Recent Eisenmenger targeted therapy studies

Author/Date	Study Type/Participants	Comments
Phosphodiesterase type 5 inhibitors (PDE-5i)		
Mukhopadhyay et al,[40] 2011	Randomized, double-blind crossover trial in 28 pts with ES on tadalafil vs placebo	• Tadalafil well tolerated • Improved 6MWD and SO(2) • Improved functional class • Decreased PVR • No change in SVR
Zhang et al,[43] 2011	Multicenter prospective open-label study in China on 84 pts with ES on sildenafil 20 mg tid for 12 mo	• Improved 6MWD • Improved SO(2) • Decreased PAP, PVR
Sun et al,[44] 2013	Retrospective review in 121 pts with ES of which 53 pts were on sildenafil	• 97, 95% survival in sildenafil group at 1, 3 y • 90, 83% survival in no treatment group at 1,3 y • Multivariate analysis of sildenafil group; FC and mPAP independently associated with survival
Endothelin receptor antagonists (ERAs):		

Zuckerman et al,[45] 2011	Retrospective review of 17 pts with ES on ambrisentan; followed short term (163 ± 57 d) and long term 2.5 ± 0.5 y	• Short term
		  ○ Improved 6MWD
		 • Long term
		  ○ No clinical deterioration

Actelion Ltd[46]	Phase III study Open-label extension in pts with ES MAESTRO and MAESTRO-OL	• Investigating effect of Opsumit (macitentan) on ES • Completion date February 2016 • SERAPHIN trial, 10 mg Opsumit reduced relative risk of morbidity and mortality in pts with PH with WHO FC II and III by 45%
Combination therapy: PDE5i and ERA:		
D'Alto et al,[47] 2012	32 pts with ES deteriorating on bosentan who then added sildenafil 20 mg tid	• 28/32 RHC due to clinical deterioration • 6 mo follow-up combo was well tolerated • Improved SO(2) and 6MWD • Increased PBF and decreased PVR
Diller et al,[48] 2012	Retrospective review of 79 pts with ES	Improvement in 6MWD with therapy escalation
Prostanoids: Selexipag		

Actelion Ltd[49]	Ongoing subanalysis of 110 PAH Pts with CHD from the GRIPHON randomized, multicenter, double-blind, placebo-controlled trial	• GRIPHON trial
		  ○ Largest outcome trial done in PAH
		  ○ 1156 pts in 181 centers in 39 countries
		  ○ Decreased risk of morbidity/mortality vs placebo by 40% over 4.3 y

Abbreviations: 6MWD, 6-minute walk distance; ES, Eisenmenger syndrome; FC, functional class; MAESTRO, macitentan on exercise capacity in subjects with eisenmenger syndrome; MAESTRO-OL, clinical study to assess the long-term safety, tolerability, and efficacy of macitentan in subjects with eisenmenger syndrome; mPAP, mean pulmonary arterial pressure; PAP, pulmonary arterial pressures; PBF, pulmonary blood flow; PH, pulmonary hypertension; pts, patients; PVR, pulmonary vascular resistance; RHC, right heart catheterization; SERAPHIN, study with an endothelin receptor antagonist in pulmonary arterial hypertension to improve clinical outcome; SO(2), systemic arterial blood oxygenation; SVR, systemic vascular resistance; tid, 3 times a day; WHO, World Health Organization.

SUMMARY

As the prevalence of ACHD continues to accelerate, a significant number of ACHDs have or will eventually develop PAH, requiring multidisciplinary care anchored by innovative medical and interventional strategies. Unique cohorts, including Down syndrome, pregnancy, and single ventricles, palliated with total cavopulmonary anastomoses add additional challenges to this complex group. Borderline hemodynamics in unrepaired or residual defects continue to challenge our treatment algorithms with management specific to institutional experience. Additional research in this subgroup is needed to better understand efficacy of targeted therapies and the safety of defect closure. Although more extensively studied, ES remains a highly debilitating disease with increased morbidity and mortality. Over the past decade, patients with ES treated with targeted PAH therapies have reliably demonstrated improvements in functional capacity, hemodynamics, and quality of life. Despite these welcoming advances, data evaluating their survival outcome are scarce. Those who fail escalating therapies are ultimately considered for transplantation, but again these results are mixed. Optimizing the care of the patient with PAH-CHD demands a comprehensive approach integrating tertiary-level resources with multicenter initiatives to best investigate the potential of contemporary medical, catheter-based, and surgical treatments.

REFERENCES

1. Marelli AJ, Therrien J, Mackie AS, et al. Planning the specialized care of adult congenital heart disease patients: from numbers to guidelines; an epidemiologic approach. Am Heart J 2009;157:1–8.

2. Engelfriet PM, Duffels MG, Möller T, et al. Pulmonary arterial hypertension in adults born with a heart septal defect: the Euro Heart Survey on adult congenital heart disease. Heart 2007;93: 682–7.

3. McLaughlin VV, Archer SL, Badesch DB, et al. ACCF/AHA 2009 expert consensus document on pulmonary hypertension a report of the American College of Cardiology Foundation Task Force on Expert Consensus Documents and the American Heart Association developed in collaboration with the American College of Chest Physicians; American Thoracic Society, Inc.; and the Pulmonary Hypertension Association. J Am Coll Cardiol 2009; 53(17):1573–619.

4. Diller GP, Gatzoulis MA. Pulmonary vascular disease in adults with congenital heart disease. Circulation 2007;115(8):1039–50.

5. Beghetti M, Galie N. Eisenmenger syndrome: a clinical perspective in a new therapeutic era of pulmonary arterial hypertension [review]. J Am Coll Cardiol 2009;53:733–40.

6. Hoeper M, Bogaard HJ, Condliffe R, et al. Definitions and diagnosis of pulmonary hypertension. J Am Coll Cardiol 2013;62(25 Suppl):D42–50.

7. Simonneau G, Gatzoulis MA, Adatia I, et al. Updated clinical classification of pulmonary hypertension. J Am Coll Cardiol 2013;62(25 Suppl):D34–41.

8. Dufflels MG, Engelfriet PM, Berger RM, et al. Pulmonary arterial hypertension in congenital heart disease; an epidemiologic perspective from a Dutch Registry. Int J Cardiol 2007;120:198–204.

9. Baumgartner H, Bonhoeffer P, De Groot NM, et al, Task Force on the Management of Grown-up Congenital Heart Disease of the European Society of Cardiology (ESC), Association for European Pediatric Cardiology (AEPC), ESC Committee for Practice Guidelines (CPG). ESC guidelines for the management of grown-up congenital heart disease (new version 2010). Eur Heart J 2010;31: 2915–57.

10. Heath D, Edwards J. The pathology of hypertensive pulmonary vascular disease. Circulation 1958;18: 533–47.

11. Wood P. The Eisenmenger syndrome or pulmonary hypertension with reversed central shunt. Br Med J 1958;2(5099):755–62.

12. Adatia I, Kothari SS, Feinstein JA. Pulmonary hypertension associated with congenital heart disease: pulmonary vascular disease: the global perspective. Chest 2010;137(6 Suppl):52S–61S.

13. Kiefer, Bashore T. Anatomy of congenital heart disease lesions associated with pulmonary arterial hypertension. Adv Pulm Hypertens 2013;11(4):166–70.

14. Vogel M, Berger F, Kramer A, et al. Incidence of secondary pulmonary hypertension in adults with atrial septal or sinus venosus defects. Heart 1999; 82:30–3.

15. Healey JE Jr. An anatomic survey of anomalous pulmonary veins: their clinical significance. J Thorac Surg 1952;23(5):433–44.

16. Waldhausen JA. The early history of congenital heart surgery: closed heart operations. Ann Thorac Surg 1997;64(5):1533–9.

17. Yoshibayashi M, Nishioka K. Plasma endothelin concentrations in patients with pulmonary hypertension associated with congenital heart defects. Evidence for increased production of endothelin in pulmonary circulation. Circulation 1991;84:2280–5.

18. Cacoub P, Dorent R, Maistre G, et al. Endothelin-1 in primary pulmonary hypertension and the Eisenmenger syndrome. Am J Cardiol 1993;71: 448–50.

19. Fratz S, Geiger R, Kresse H, et al. Pulmonary blood pressure, not flow, is associated with net

endothelin-1 production in the lungs of patients with congenital heart disease and normal pulmonary vascular resistance. J Thorac Cardiovasc Surg 2003;126(6):1724–9.

20. Moceri P, Kempny A, Liodakis E, et al. Physiologic differences between various types of Eisenmenger syndrome and relation to outcome. Int J Cardiol 2015;179:455–60.

21. Alonso-Gonzalez R, Lopez-Guarch CJ, Subirana-Domenech MT, et al. Pulmonary hypertension and congenital heart disease: an insight from the REHAP National Registry. Int J Cardiol 2015;184:717–23.

22. Kidd L, Driscoll DJ, Gersony WM, et al. Second natural history study of congenital heart defects. Results of treatment of patients with ventricular septal defects. Circulation 1993; 87(2 Suppl):I38–51.

23. Steele PM, Fuster V, Cohen M, et al. Isolated atrial septal defect with pulmonary vascular obstructive disease long-term follow-up and prediction of outcome after surgical correction. Circulation 1987; 76(5):1037–42.

24. Moceri P, Dimopoulos K, Liodakis E, et al. Echocardiographic predictors of outcome in Eisenmenger syndrome. Circulation 2012;126:1461–8.

25. van Riel AC, Schuuring MJ, van Hessen ID, et al. Contemporary prevalence of pulmonary arterial hypertension in adult congenital heart disease following the updated clinical classification. Int J Cardiol 2014;174:299–305.

26. Chan E, Alejos J. Pulmonary hypertension in patients after repair of transposition of the great arteries. Congenit Heart Dis 2010;5(2):161–4.

27. Cordina R, Celermajer D. Late-onset pulmonary arterial hypertension after a successful atrial or arterial switch procedure for transposition of the great arteries. Pediatr Cardiol 2010;31(2):238–41.

28. Dimopoulos K, Wort SJ, Gatzoulis MA. Pulmonary hypertension related to congenital heart disease; a call for action. Eur Heart J 2014;35:691–700.

29. Rosenkranz S, Ghofrani HA, Beghetti M, et al. Riociguat for pulmonary arterial hypertension associated with congenital heart disease. Heart 2015;101(22): 1792–9.

30. Stellin G, Vida VL, Padalino MA, European Congenital Heart Surgeons Association. Surgical outcome for congenital heart malformations in the adult age: a multicentric European study. Semin Thorac Cardiovasc Surg Pediatr Card Surg Annu 2004;7:95–101.

31. Hoffman JI, Kaplan S. The incidence of congenital heart disease. J Am Coll Cardiol 2002;39(12): 1890–900.

32. Aboulhosn J, Levi D, Moore J. Transcatheter interventions in adults with congenital heart disease. In: Perloff JK, Child J, Aboulhosn J, editors. Congenital heart disease in adults. 3rd edition. Philadelphia: Saunders; 2008.

33. Aboulhonsn JA. The role of catheter-based and surgical treatments in patients with congenital heart disease and pulmonary hypertension. Adv Pulm Hypertens 2013;11(4):189–94.

34. Mahan G, Dabestani A, Gardin J, et al. Estimation of pulmonary artery pressure by pulsed Doppler echocardiography. Circulation 1983;68:367.

35. Kaul S, Tei C, Hopkins JM, et al. Assessment of right ventricular function using two-dimensional echocardiography. Am Heart J 1984;107(3):526–31.

36. Ghio S, Klersy C, Magrini G, et al. Prognostic relevance of the echocardiographic assessment of right ventricular function in patients with idiopathic pulmonary arterial hypertension. Int J Cardiol 2010;140(3): 272–8.

37. Manes A, Palazzini M, Leci E, et al. Current era survival of patients with pulmonary arterial hypertension associated with congenital heart disease: a comparison between clinical subgroups. Eur Heart J 2014; 35:716–24.

38. Inai K. Can pulmonary vasodilator therapy expand the operative indications for congenital heart disease. Int Heart J 2015;56:S12–6.

39. D'Alto M, Romeo E, Argiento P, et al. Hemodynamics of patients developing pulmonary arterial hypertension after shunt closure. Int J Cardiol 2013;168: 3797–801.

40. Mukhopadhyay S, Nathani S, Yusuf J, et al. Clinical efficacy of phosphodiesterase-5 inhibitor tadalafil in Eisenmenger syndrome–a randomized, placebo-controlled, double-blind crossover study. Congenit Heart Dis 2011;6:424–31.

41. Warnes CA, Williams RG, Bashore TM, et al. ACC/AHA 2008 guidelines for the management of adults with congenital heart disease: a report of the American College of Cardiology/American Heart Association Task Force on Practice Guidelines (writing committee to develop guidelines on the management of adults with congenital heart disease). Circulation 2008;118(23):e714–833.

42. Galie N, Beghetti M, Gatzoulis MA, et al. Bosentan therapy in patients with Eisenmenger syndrome; a multicenter, double-blind, randomized placebo-controlled study. Circulation 2006;114(1):48–54.

43. Zhang ZN, Jiang X, Zhang R, et al. Oral sildenafil treatment for Eisenmenger syndrome: a prospective, open-label, multicentre study. Heart 2011;97: 1876–81.

44. Sun YJ, Yang T, Zeng WJ, et al. Impact of sildenafil on survival of patients with Eisenmenger syndrome. J Clin Pharmacol 2013;53:611–8.

45. Zuckerman WA, Leaderer D, Rowan CA, et al. Ambrisentan for pulmonary arterial hypertension due to congenital heart disease. Am J Cardiol 2011;107(9):1381–5.

46. Available at: https://www.clinicaltrials.gov/ct2/show/NCT01739400.

47. D'Alto M, Romeo E, Argiento P, et al. Bosentan-sildenafil association in patients with congenital heart disease-related pulmonary arterial hypertension and Eisenmenger physiology. Int J Cardiol 2012; 155:378–82.

48. Diller GP, Alonso-Gonzalez R, Dimopoulos K, et al. Disease targeting therapies in patients with Eisenmenger syndrome: response to treatment and long-term efficiency. Int J Cardiol 2012;167: 840–7.

49. Available at: https://www.clinicaltrials.gov/ct2/show/NCT01106014.

50. Karamlou T, Hirsch J, Welke K, et al. A United Network for Organ Sharing analysis of heart transplantation in adults with congenital heart disease: outcomes and factors associated with mortality and retransplantation. J Thorac Cardiovasc Surg 2010;140(1):161–8.

51. Choong CK, Sweet SC, Guthrie TJ, et al. Repair of congenital heart lesions combined with lung transplantation for the treatment of severe pulmonary hypertension: a 13-year experience. J Thorac Cardiovasc Surg 2005;129(3):661–9.

52. Everitt MD, Donaldson AE, Stehlik J, et al. Would access to device therapies improve transplant outcomes for adults with congenital heart disease? Analysis of the United Network for Organ Sharing (UNOS). J Heart Lung Transplant 2011; 30(4):395–401.

53. Russo P, Wheeler A, Russo J, et al. Use of a ventricular assist device as a bridge to transplantation in a patient with single ventricle physiology and total cavopulmonary anastomosis. Paediatr Anaesth 2008;18(4):320.

54. Alphonso N, Baghai M, Sundar P, et al. Intermediate-term outcome following the Fontan operation: a survival, functional and risk-factor analysis. Eur J Cardiothorac Surg 2005;28:529–35.

55. Derk G, Houser L, Miner P, et al. Efficacy of endothelin blockade in adults with Fontan physiology. Congenit Heart Dis 2015;10(1):E11–6.

56. Giardini A, Balducci A, Specchia S, et al. Effect of sildenafil on haemodynamic response to exercise and exercise capacity in Fontan patients. Eur Heart J 2008;29:1681–7.

57. Goldberg DJ, French B, McBride MG, et al. Impact of oral sildenafil on exercise performance in children and young adults after the Fontan operation: a randomized, double blind, placebo-controlled, crossover trial. Circulation 2011;123:1185–93.

58. Schuuring MJ, Vis JC, van Dijk APJ, et al. Impact of bosentan on exercise capacity in adults after the Fontan procedure: a randomized controlled trial. Eur J Heart Fail 2013;15:690–8.

59. Herbet A, Mikkelsen UR, Thilen U, et al. Bosentan improves exercise capacity in adolescents and adults after Fontan operation: the TEMPO (Treatment With Endothelin Receptor Antagonist in Fontan Patients, a Randomized, Placebo-Controlled, Double-Blind Study Measuring Peak Oxygen Consumption) study. Circulation 2014;130(23):2021–30.

Group 2 Pulmonary Hypertension
Pulmonary Venous Hypertension: Epidemiology and Pathophysiology

Craig B. Clark, DO[a], Evelyn M. Horn, MD[b],*

KEYWORDS

- Pulmonary hypertension • Left heart disease • Valvular disease • Epidemiology • Pathophysiology

KEY POINTS

- Pulmonary hypertension from left heart disease (PH-LHD) is a common form of pulmonary hypertension.
- PH-LHD occurs secondary to left ventricular systolic dysfunction, diastolic dysfunction, and/or left-sided valvular disease, which increases left atrial pressure that is transmitted backward to the pulmonary veins, capillaries, and arteries.
- In addition to the passive transmission of left atrial pressure to the pulmonary circulation, some patients develop superimposed precapillary pulmonary vascular pathology.
- Prognosis in PH-LHD is related to right ventricular function.
- No disease-specific therapies currently exist.

INTRODUCTION

Pulmonary hypertension (PH) induced by left-sided heart disease (PH-LHD) or Group 2 PH is the most prevalent PH form.[1–3] It is seen in heart failure (HF) with reduced ejection fraction (HFrEF), HF with preserved ejection fraction (HFpEF), and significant left-sided valvular disease. PH-LHD remains a major challenge for the clinician when faced with a dyspneic patient who exhibits an elevated pulmonary artery systolic pressure (PASP) (typically discovered on echo) to determine whether their patient has PH-LHD because treatment differs markedly from other forms of PH.

Despite its prevalence, PH-LHD has only recently been a focus for interventions; as yet, effective treatment strategies have not been established beyond addressing the treatment of the underlying left heart disease. We review

mechanisms involved in the pathophysiologic development of PH-LHD and its consequences of right ventricular (RV) failure, discuss hemodynamic testing to both aid in diagnosis as well as to better understand the pathophysiology, briefly touch on the limited treatment options, and address future research areas.

DEFINITIONS

In addition to the commonly referred to World Health Organization (WHO) Group 2 classification, PH-LHD has had multiple, sometimes confusing descriptors in the literature, often without clear hemodynamic criteria, making it challenging to characterize, compare, and study. Terminologies that have been used to address PH-LHD include pulmonary venous hypertension, mechanical versus active PH, out-of-proportion PH, passive

No relevant conflict of interests to disclose.
[a] Division of Cardiology, Department of Internal Medicine, Des Moines University, Iowa Heart Center, Des Moines, IA 50312, USA; [b] Division of Cardiology, Perkin Heart Failure Center, Weill Cornell Medical Center, 520 East 70th Street, Starr Pavilion, 4th Floor, New York, NY 10021, USA
* Corresponding author.
E-mail address: horneve@med.cornell.edu

Cardiol Clin 34 (2016) 401–411
http://dx.doi.org/10.1016/j.ccl.2016.04.010
0733-8651/16/$ – see front matter © 2016 Elsevier Inc. All rights reserved.

versus reactive, and mixed PH. This heterogeneity stems from the complex nature of PH-LHD, which begins as an increased left atrial or pulmonary venous pressure that is passively transmitted backward proximal to the pulmonary venous system, that is, pulmonary capillaries and pulmonary arteries. For reasons not fully understood, a segment of patients will go on to develop superimposed pulmonary vascular disease, that is, an elevated transpulmonary gradient (TPG) and/or diastolic pulmonary gradient (DPG) and elevated pulmonary vascular resistance (PVR), exhibiting clinical hemodynamic characteristics of precapillary pulmonary arterial hypertension (PAH), defined as follows.

To bring consistency, the 5th World Symposium on PH (WSPH) endorsed the nomenclature "isolated post-capillary PH" (iso-PH) and "combined post-capillary and precapillary PH" (Cpc-PH) based on characteristic hemodynamic profiles and to abandon the term "out-of-proportion" PH.[4] Thus, PH-LHD is defined as mean pulmonary artery pressure (mPAP) of 25 mm Hg or higher with a pulmonary artery wedge pressure (PAWP) of greater than 15 mm Hg.[5] An elevated DPG is defined as follows: diastolic pulmonary artery pressure (PAP)-PAWP of greater than 7 mm Hg identifies Cpc-PH and separates it from iso-PH,[4] although this classification has not been without controversy.[6] An elevated TPG, defined as mPAP minus PAWP greater than 12 to 15 mm Hg, and elevated PVR, defined as TPG/cardiac output greater than 3 WU, have previously been used to describe "out-of-proportion" PH-LHD,[7] and remain useful parameters in the overall hemodynamic assessment of patients with PH. However, because they are influenced by flow and by left atrial pressure, DPG has been advocated as the metric of choice to differentiate iso-PH from Cpc-PH, as it is relatively unaffected by flow or filling pressures and should therefore more precisely represent the independent contribution of the pulmonary vasculature to PAP.[4,8]

PH-LHD is often initially identified not by invasive pressure measurement at catheterization but by echocardiography, where mPAP is typically not calculated and instead PASP is estimated from tricuspid regurgitation Doppler velocity added to an estimate of right atrial (RA) pressure, typically gleaned from IVC (inferior vena cava) diameter. In this situation, a PASP of 35 to 45 mm Hg is typically considered mildly elevated, whereas 46 to 60 mm Hg and greater than 60 mm Hg are considered moderately elevated and severely elevated, respectively.[9] Although Doppler echocardiography has proven to be an excellent screening tool, cardiac catheterization is required for definitive diagnosis and is mandatory before instituting PH-specific therapies. Furthermore, many echocardiology laboratories fail to report systemic blood pressures to better assess PASP in relation to systemic pressures.

EPIDEMIOLOGY

Due to variabilities in PH definitions with predominant echo-based literature data and referral bias,[10] the true prevalence is likely underappreciated.[11] In 379 consecutive patients with HFrEF undergoing right heart catheterization (RHC), Ghio and colleagues[12] found PH, defined as mPAP greater than 20 mm Hg at catheterization, in 62%. Its presence correlated with more advanced disease manifest by New York Heart Association class III/IV symptoms, lower CO, and lower RV EF. However, the development of PH does not directly correlate with the degree of left ventricular (LV) EF reduction.[13] In fact, HFpEF has been recognized as the predominant cause of PH-LHD.[14] In an echo-Doppler study of patients with HFpEF, PH defined as an estimated PASP greater than 35 mm Hg, was identified in 83%, whereas in a comparative community cohort of patients with hypertension without HF, it was present in only 8%.[10] In a random sample of the general population from Olmsted County, Minnesota, elevated echo-estimated PASP correlated with increasing age, systemic vascular stiffness as assessed by brachial artery pulse pressure, and elevated left heart diastolic pressure inferred from echo-Doppler E/e' ratio.[15] In other studies, elevated echo-estimated PASP was seen more frequently in patients with obesity, atrial arrhythmias, and chronic obstructive pulmonary disease (COPD),[16] all common comorbidities associated with the HFpEF syndrome but that also may be independent pathophysiological causative factors of PH. In patients with PH-LHD, the presence of Cpc-PH has varied depending on the population studied, ranging from 12% to more than 50%, with similar frequencies between HFrEF and HFpEF.[17–19] A recent study by Gerges and colleagues[19] showed that Cpc-PH was present in only 12% of patients: HFpEF and HFrEF in retrospective and prospective cohorts. Risk factors differed in HFpEF and HFrEF for Cpc-PH. Whereas COPD and echo ratio of TAPSE/PASP were associated in the patients with systolic HF, younger age, VHD and TAPSE/PASP were associated with Cpc-PH in the patients with diastolic HF. RV/pulmonary artery (PA) coupling (Ees/Ea) is worse in all patients with Cpc-PH. Given the aging population and increasing burden of HF, particularly that of HFpEF, the incidence of PH-LHD can be expected to rise.[20]

In patients with valvular heart disease, the development of PH is a marker of severity[2] and should be an indication to consider intervention. However, its presence also can be associated with a higher risk of procedural morbidity. According to one study, 10% to 15% of patients older than 75 years have moderate to severe valvular dysfunction, affecting equal numbers of men and women.[21] Nearly all patients with symptomatic mitral valve disease have some degree of PH[2] with moderate or severe PH present in 24% of those with mitral stenosis and 27% with mitral regurgitation.[22] In mitral regurgitation, the presence of PH is directly associated with the severity of the mitral regurgitation,[23] and in patients with LV systolic dysfunction who also have functional mitral regurgitation, PH is found in 40%.[22] Following mitral valve surgery there is often a rapid reduction in PA pressures, representing resolution of the iso-PH component as left atrial pressure normalizes. However, in patients with Cpc-PH from pulmonary vascular remodeling, reduction in PA pressures and PVR may take months or improve only partially.[24]

In aortic valve disease, PH correlates with LV and/or atrial dysfunction. Johnson and colleagues[25] found PH, defined as catheter-derived PASP greater than 30 mm Hg, in 50% of their patients with severe aortic stenosis (AS) referred for valve replacement. In their cohort, severe PH (PASP >50 mm Hg) was present in 16%. Silver and colleagues[26] reported PH (catheter-derived PASP >50 mm Hg) in 29% of symptomatic patients with severe AS. Those with PH had more clinical HF, lower LV ejection fraction, lower cardiac index, and more MR (mitral regurgitation). Similarly, with severe aortic regurgitation, PH was found in 24% and correlated with elevated LV end-diastolic pressure.[27] In an older population referred for transcutaneous aortic valve replacement (TAVR), prevalence of PH is significantly higher and long-term outcomes post intervention poorer. PASP greater than 40 mm Hg by echocardiography was associated with a higher 1-year but not 30-day mortality.[28] This was especially so in patients with severe PH defined as a PASP greater than 60 mm Hg.[28] However, patients whose PASP decreased to less than 60 mm Hg following TAVR did significantly better than those with persistently severe PH at 2 years.[29]

New insights into PH-LHD may come from remote telemonitoring via implantable PA pressure sensors. In a substudy of the CHAMPION trial evaluating a wireless, implantable hemodynamic monitoring device, 49% of patients who did not have PH at baseline went on to exhibit PH during their first week of monitoring, suggesting that PH-LHD is underdiagnosed even in a group known to be at high risk.[11]

Several studies have demonstrated increased morbidity and mortality associated with PH-LHD. Bursi and colleagues[13] found that echo-derived elevated PASP in a community cohort of patients with HFrEF and HFpEF was associated with an increased mortality. In CHAMPION, patients with PH had higher mortality and readmission rates. Hemodynamically guided outpatient management reduced hospitalizations but did not impact survival.[30] Comparing outcomes between patients with HFrEF and HFpEF with PH, Salamon and colleagues[31] found higher 5-year mortality in the HFpEF group.

Despite these data, the question remains whether PH is itself a risk factor for poor outcomes, a marker of more advanced disease and/or summation of comorbidities and ultimately, whether it is a target for intervention. Miller and colleagues[32] found that in matched cohorts of patients with HFrEF, echo-Doppler–derived PASP greater than 45 mm Hg was a marker of all-cause mortality that was independent of other variables, including LV dysfunction or functional mitral regurgitation. Much of the morbidity and mortality associated with PH-LHD appears related to the development of RV failure.[19,32,33] Unfortunately, trials to date specifically targeting PH have shown no improvements in outcomes.[24] However, these studies took all comers with PH and did not specifically target those with Cpc-PH. More data are needed to define whether PH is, in fact, an independent therapeutic target in specific patient cohorts with left-sided heart disease.

COMMON PATHOPHYSIOLOGIC MECHANISMS IN PULMONARY HYPERTENSION INDUCED BY LEFT-SIDED HEART DISEASE

The primary driver of the post-capillary process in PH-LHD is an elevated left atrial pressure, which is transmitted backward to the pulmonary venous system, pulmonary capillaries, and ultimately to the pulmonary arteries. In iso-PH characterized by an elevated PAP but with a low diastolic pressure gradient (PAD-PAWP <7 mm Hg), normal PVR (<3 WU), and normal TPG (<12 mm Hg) there remains a "normal" pulmonary vascular response, although histologically, abnormalities such as intimal fibrosis and medial hypertrophy may already be developing.[34,35]

Elevated left atrial pressure most commonly originates from elevated LV diastolic pressure due to systolic or diastolic dysfunction. However, in mitral valve disease, as with the noncompliant left atrial syndrome, LV pressure may be normal. Furthermore, functional mitral regurgitation, intrinsic left atrium (LA) disease (such as LA myopathy and/or fibrosis), and atrial arrhythmias play important roles in the development of PH-LHD. These processes lead to inefficient atrial emptying and loss of atrial compliance, which increases LA and thus pulmonary venous pressure. Changes in the pulmonary veins, capillaries, and arteries may develop, further potentiating the problem so that the normally high-capacitance, low-resistance pulmonary vascular circuit (with a fixed RC (resistance-compliance) coupling relationship) is shifted such that pulmonary arterial compliance is less for a given resistance. This "stiff" pulmonary vasculature creates a disproportionately elevated pulsatile RV load (relative to a resistive load), thereby increasing RV work, promoting RV dysfunction, and ultimately leading to right HF.[19,36,37]

A subset of patients with PH-LHD develop superimposed precapillary pulmonary arterial disease with vasoconstriction and vascular remodeling that increases PVR, further elevating PAP beyond that which is generated by backward transmission of LA hypertension alone. This has been referred to as "fixed" or "reactive" pulmonary vascular disease, and more recently descriptively termed "combined post-capillary and precapillary pulmonary hypertension" (Cpc-PH). It is characterized by an elevated DPG greater than 7 mm Hg, an elevated PVR of greater than 3 WU, and elevated TPG greater than 12 to 15 mm Hg that may be fixed or reversible.[4,5]

The following sections address these processes in more detail.

The Left Atrium

A detailed discussion of LV dysfunction and the pathophysiology of HFrEF and HFpEF is beyond the scope of this article and the reader is referred to some excellent reviews in the literature.[38,39] We begin our discussion with the left atrium.

Two well-described phenomena relate to left atrial dysfunction that may play a role in PH-LHD: (1) Pilote and colleagues[40] and Mehta and colleagues[41] described the "stiff left atrial syndrome" in the 1980s/1990s; and (2) the loss of atrial contraction due to the development of atrial fibrillation reduces stroke volume and can precipitate decompensation in patients with HF or mitral stenosis. Despite these phenomena described years ago, the role of left atrial dysfunction in HF, particularly in PH-LHD has not been well studied. It is increasingly appreciated that the LA is more than simply a passive conduit and that primary disease of the LA, which may be associated with atrial and ventricular myocardial fibrosis, leads to structural

changes that contribute importantly to the development of PH and right-sided HF[42] as well as to thrombogenic risk in atrial fibrillation. Melenovsky and colleagues[42] showed that chronically increased left atrial preloads and afterloads seen in both HFrEF and HFpEF lead to the development of left atrial remodeling with progressive enlargement and stiffness. They showed that HFrEF was associated with more eccentric remodeling and greater LA enlargement, whereas in HFpEF, the LA becomes stiffer and has a greater propensity to develop atrial fibrillation. Both HFrEF and HFpEF are associated with LA contractile dysfunction, but to a greater extent in HFrEF.[42] As expected, these changes correlate with the presence of PH and RV dysfunction. Furthermore, left atrial contractile function is inversely related to PVR and directly related to RV systolic function.[42]

Interestingly, left atrial remodeling mirrors that seen with the LV in HFrEF and HFpEF, suggesting that the LA's remodeling response may be influenced by the company it keeps. Whereas a dilated cardiomyopathy may directly affect the LA as well as the LV and lead to greater eccentric remodeling, conditions associated with ventricular stiffness in HFpEF; for example, long-standing hypertension, diabetes, obesity, vascular stiffness, and chronic kidney disease, may similarly affect the left atrium.[39] The comorbidities of HFpEF also produce a systemic proinflammatory state, further contributing to microvascular endothelial dysfunction, vasoconstrictor/vasodilator imbalance, hypertrophy, and fibrosis.[43,44] Patients with atrial fibrillation often develop a fibrotic atrial cardiomyopathy, and inflammation has been similarly implicated in its pathogenesis.[45,46] As atrial fibrillation is seen more frequently in HFpEF,[39] common mechanisms may be involved in the development of these 2 disease processes. Angiotensin II and transforming growth factor beta-1 (TGF-B1) are the most potent stimulators of collagen synthesis.[47,48] In transgenic mice with TGF-B1 overexpression, upregulation was more pronounced in the atria leading to the development of isolated atrial fibrosis. However, when TGF-B1 overexpression was coupled with other pathophysiologic stimuli of HF, fibrosis was enhanced in the ventricles as well.[49]

The Pulmonary Veins and Capillaries

Pulmonary arterial remodeling is known to occur in PH-LHD, particularly in Cpc-PH; however, vascular changes may also occur at the level of the pulmonary veins and capillaries. These changes, particularly at the capillary level, precede those of arterial remodeling.[7] "Arterialization" of the pulmonary veins has been described in response to chronically elevated LA pressure, with increased vessel wall thickness due to the development of double elastic laminae and hypertrophy of the medial layer. The degree of intimal, medial, and adventitial remodeling is akin to that seen in the pulmonary arteries.[50,51]

Elevated pulmonary venous pressure is transmitted upstream to the pulmonary capillaries. An acute increase in intracapillary pressure can disrupt the delicate alveolar-capillary membrane, causing fracturing and leading to alveolar-capillary stress failure.[52] But when the pressure increase occurs more slowly, adaptive changes develop in the congested capillaries, venules, and arterioles. This chronic pressure elevation induces a multitude of neurohormonal and biochemical sequences giving rise to activation of growth factors resulting in remodeling, hypertrophy, and fibrosis with deposition of type IV collagen into the basal lamina, increasing alveolar-capillary membrane thickness.[53] With elevated pulmonary venous pressure, focal thickening of alveolar septa develops and lung tissue fibroblast proliferation leads to deposition of elastin and reticular fibrils.[54] These changes may protect against the development of pulmonary edema, but they impair gas exchange and contribute to the sensation of dyspnea. Altered gene expression of extracellular matrix proteins and platelet-derived growth factor-B induced by increased intracapillary pressure and alveolar hypoxia from impaired gas exchange, may lead to chronic remodeling changes.[55]

The Pulmonary Arteries

Pulmonary artery remodeling in PH-LHD has similarities to WHO group 1 PAH but is less severe and is without characteristic plexogenic lesions.[24] Medial hypertrophy is the most prominent pathologic finding.[56] Smooth muscle cell growth and migration are activated through the induction of endogenous vascular serine elastase, the release of growth factors, and of glycoproteins.[2,7,57,58] Intimal fibrosis also develops and is often extensive and severe.[59] This may be accompanied by intimal edema resulting from pulmonary venous congestion.[53] These structural changes increase PVR and impede the vasculature's ability to respond to acute vasodilator testing. However, with sustained hemodynamic improvement after LV assist device or cardiac transplantation, partial reversibility remains.[60]

Similar to WHO Group 1 PH, imbalanced vasodilator and vasoconstrictor substances, most notably nitric oxide (NO) and endothelin-1 (ET1) along with a blunted response to the natriuretic peptides contribute to endothelial dysfunction.[61] ET1 is elevated in chronic HF and its level correlates with both PA pressure[62] and mortality.[63] Other mediators of HF, such as catecholamines, angiotensin II, and aldosterone, are likely also involved in generating a chronic vasoconstricted state. Importantly, despite endothelial dysfunction, the vasculature still exhibits a reversible response on acute vasodilator testing with reduction of PAP and narrowing of the TPG, as long as vascular remodeling is not too extensive.

These changes in the pulmonary arteries are paramount to the development of PH-LHD and particularly important in the transition from iso-PH to Cpc-PH.

Given their central roles, the NO and ET1 pathways have been targets for therapy in HF and PH-LHD. Unfortunately, favorable acute hemodynamic responses have not translated into improved outcomes.[24,64] Sildenafil is a phosphodiesterase-5 inhibitor that prevents degradation of cyclic guanosine monophosphate (cGMP) enhancing NO-dependent vasodilation in the lungs without significantly effecting systemic circulation. In addition to its vasodilating properties, sildenafil has antiproliferative effects,[65] potentiates natriuretic peptides,[66] and favorably impacts RV function.[67,68] It seemingly would be an ideal therapy in PH-LHD. The RELAX (Evaluating the Effectiveness of Sildenafil at Improving Health Outcomes and Exercise Ability in People with Diastolic Heart Failure) trial, however, failed to show any benefit in a group of symptomatic HFpEF patients, although PH was not a prespecified entry criterion.[69]

A related compound, Riociguat, an oral soluble guanylate cyclase stimulator approved for WHO Groups 1 and 4 PH, was evaluated in the DILATE-1 (A Study to Test the Effects of Riociguat in Patients with Pulmonary Hypertension Associated With Left Ventricular Diastolic Dysfunction) trial. Although well tolerated, a single 2-mg dose showed no effect on mPAP, heart rate, PAWP, TPG, or PVR. Reductions were seen in RV end diastolic area, systemic vascular resistance (SVR), and systemic blood pressure with an associated increase in stroke volume.[70] A phase IIB study in PH associated with LV systolic dysfunction (LEPHT) showed an increase in cardiac index and reductions in PVR and SVR at the 2-mg dose but failed to reach its primary endpoint of a reduction in mPAP.[71] Furthermore, concern was raised that although thermodilution cardiac index increased, mixed venous oxygen saturation did not. In addition, there was no improvement in exercise capacity.[72]

Various ET1 receptor antagonists (ERAs) have been studied in both acute and chronic HFrEF. Despite promising early results, no outcome improvements have been demonstrated, and some studies have shown worsening HF requiring hospitalization[64] as well as elevations of hepatic function tests.[73]

It is noteworthy that pulmonary vascular changes in patients with PH-LHD remain highly variable despite similar degrees of pulmonary venous hypertension, suggesting a genetic predisposition to pulmonary vascular remodeling.[74] Polymorphisms of the serotonin transporter gene have been associated with smooth muscle cell dysfunction, vasoconstriction, and remodeling. Patients with HFrEF with the homozygous long variant (LL) phenotype demonstrate higher PA pressures.[75]

The Right Ventricle

The RV differs embryonically and structurally from the LV, originating from distinct precursor cells termed the anterior heart field. The RV has thinner walls, a lower mass, and a crescentic shape. It is made up of a deep longitudinal muscular layer and a superficial circumferential layer that is continuous with myofibrils of the LV.[76] This is contrasted with the LV, which originates from the primary heart field along with the atria, has thicker walls, and an elliptical shape. The LV has 3 muscular layers; a deep longitudinal layer, an oblique superficial layer, and a circular layer in between. The RV is better able to tolerate increases in volume than increases in pressure and is extremely afterload sensitive.[77] Although compensatory RV hypertrophy allows for some adaptation, eventually these mechanisms can become overwhelmed and maladaptive enlargement begins. Dilation of the tricuspid annulus leads to regurgitation, further perpetuating the process.

With PH, the shape of the RV changes from crescentic to spherical. Within a limited intrapericardial space, the shared interventricular septum shifts left as RV pressure and volume increase, impairing LV filling and reducing stroke volume.[78] Right atrial pressure increases as the RV fails, resulting in systemic venous congestion and development of an inflammatory state, as well as the development of hepatopathy, ascites, cardiorenal syndrome, and peripheral edema.

Unfortunately, the mechanisms leading from a compensated, hypertrophied RV to a dilated, failing RV are incompletely understood. Afterload mismatch, or RV-PA uncoupling, is likely the primary factor.[77] Normally, the RV's response to increased afterload is to increase contractility proportionally so that stroke volume is maintained and the RV-PA relationship remains coupled. Contractility can be represented as RV end systolic elastance (Ees). Ees is defined as the slope of the end systolic pressure-volume linear relationship. Afterload can be represented as the effective arterial elastance (Ea). Ea is defined as the change in arterial pressure for a change in volume.[77] Of note, RV afterload is often represented by its surrogate, PVR. However, PVR only reflects the restrictive component of the total pulmonary vascular load and does not account for pulsatile load, which arises from blood flow pulsatility and wave reflections through the vasculature tree. This is particularly important in PH-LHD because in post-capillary PH, unlike precapillary PH, the elevated PAWP alters pulmonary vascular compliance, creating a stiffer vasculature and thereby imposing a greater pulsatile load on the RV.[36] When the increase in contractility no longer matches the increase in afterload (Ees/Ea ratio <1), the RV-PA relationship becomes uncoupled, RV stroke volume decreases, and RV failure begins.[77]

However, beyond afterload mismatch, Melenovsky and colleagues[79] showed superimposed contractile impairment in patients with HFpEF who developed RV failure. They also showed that patients with HFrEF generally exhibit greater degrees of RV dysfunction than those with HFpEF.[79] Although an inverse relationship between RV ejection fraction and PAP has been demonstrated,[80] this relationship is extremely heterogeneous, with some patients maintaining normal RVEF in the face of PH, whereas others develop RV dysfunction despite normal PA pressures. This may be partially explained by underlying myopathic processes involving the RV as well as the LV, or inflammation and neurohormonal stimulation from the renin angiotensin aldosterone and sympathetic nervous systems contributing to RV remodeling.[81] In addition, certain patients with PH-LHD may have a genetic predisposition to develop RV failure.

There may also be processes involved in PH-LHD unique to the RV. Animal models suggest that there may be inadequate capillary density within the myocardium of failing RVs.[82] Potus and colleagues[83] showed that microRNA 126, a critical regulator of angiogenesis, was downregulated in humans with RV failure due to PAH. This along with increased RV wall stress can lead to impaired perfusion resulting in supply-demand mismatch and chronic ischemia. Changes in mitochondrial function then lead to generation of oxygen radicals, furthering inflammation, and an oxidative-stress state[84] with apoptosis. Failing myocytes shift their metabolism from fatty acid oxidation to glucose utilization, requiring less oxygen but at the expense of reduced ATP production and accumulation of lipotoxic compounds within the cytoplasm.[85] Finally, revision to fetal gene expression has been demonstrated in the RV of cats subjected to chronic pressure overload.[86]

Early work with murine models of a failing RV show that stimulation of adrenergic receptor alpha-1, subtype A, can enhance inotropy, prevent fibrosis, and reduce cell death.[87] However, although strides have been made, our understanding of the pathophysiology underlying RV dysfunction remains rudimentary, no targeted therapies exist, and much work remains to be done.

HEMODYNAMIC TESTING

Definitive diagnosis and categorization of PH-LHD requires invasive hemodynamic assessment by RHC and sometimes left heart catheterization. Careful attention must be paid to obtaining accurate measurements, in particular that of the PAWP. Recommendations made from the 5th WSPH include the following: (1) A comprehensive hemodynamic assessment should be done on every patient undergoing RHC to include RA, RV, PA and "wedge" pressures, CO via the gold standard direct Fick method or thermodilution method, and mixed-venous oxygen saturation measurement. (2) If the PA oxygen saturation exceeds 75%, full oximetry should be performed to exclude shunt. (3) Transducer zero level should be at the mid thoracic line in a supine patient halfway between the anterior sternum and the bed surface. (4) PAWP should be recorded as the mean of 3 measurements taken at end-expiration.[88] If there is question regarding the accuracy of PAWP, then a wedge oxygen saturation should be obtained or direct measurement of LV diastolic pressure performed.

The role of vasodilator testing in patients not in WHO group 1, as well as the use of provocative measures, such as volume loading or exercise to unmask occult HFpEF hemodynamics in patients with normal left-sided filling pressures at rest, is controversial.

A favorable response to a nitroprusside vasodilator challenge with reduction in PAWP, mPAP, and PVR without systemic hypotension is associated with improved mortality following heart transplantation in HFrEF.[89] The role of systemic vasodilator challenge is less clear in HFpEF when compared with HFrEF; patients experience greater

systemic blood pressure reduction and less improvement in CO despite a similar reduction in LV diastolic pressure.[17]

Differentiating WHO 1 PAH from WHO 2 in patients with normal LV function can be challenging. Further, patients treated with diuretics may exhibit normal resting left-sided filling pressures. Administration of 500 mL saline over 5 to 10 minutes has been shown safe and may be helpful in identifying occult left heart disease.[90]

Exercise also elevates filling and PA pressures in patients with left-sided heart disease and has been used in some centers along with measurement of gas exchange to perform hemodynamic cardiopulmonary exercise tests. Compared with a volume challenge, exercise during catheterization elicits greater increases in RA, PA, and PAW pressures and may have a higher sensitivity for detecting occult HFpEF.[91] Limitations of both of these methods include lack of standardized protocols and uniform definitions regarding what degree of change is physiologic versus pathologic. Recently, it has been proposed that by combining a total pulmonary resistance derived from the ratio mPAP/CO of greater than 3 WU with a maximal exercise mPAP greater than 30 mm Hg, identification of exercise-induced PH can be made with high sensitivity (93%) and greater specificity (100%). Accuracy remained high regardless of whether PH was due to pulmonary vascular disease or LHD.[92] If validated, this may become an important new methodology.

SUMMARY

PH-LHD is a common form of pulmonary hypertension and is defined as mPAP of 25 mm Hg or higher with PAWP of 15 mm Hg or higher. It begins as iso-PH originating from passive transmission of elevated pulmonary venous and/or left atrial pressure. Over time, a superimposed precapillary component can develop, and is thought to be due to vasoconstriction and structural remodeling of the pulmonary vasculature, resulting in combined post-capillary and precapillary PH that is characterized by an elevated DPG greater than 7 mm Hg. The combined effect of increased RV afterload and RV contractile dysfunction from processes just beginning to be understood lead to RV dysfunction and ultimately RV failure. The development of PH-LHD is associated with more severe left-sided disease and its presence portends a poor prognosis, particularly once RV failure develops. Treatment remains focused on the underlying left heart disease, and despite initial enthusiasm for the use of PH-specific therapies, such as prostanoids, sildenafil, and endothelin receptor blockers, studies have been disappointing and their routine clinical use cannot be recommended. More work is urgently needed to better understand the pathophysiology underlying this disease and to develop effective therapeutic strategies.

REFERENCES

1. Rosenkranz S, Gibbs JS, Wachter R, et al. Left ventricular heart failure and pulmonary hypertension. Eur Heart J 2016;37(12):942–54.

2. Wilson SR, Stefano G, Scelsi L, et al. Pulmonary hypertension and right ventricular dysfunction in left heart disease (group 2 pulmonary hypertension). Prog Cardiovasc Dis 2012;55:104–18.

3. Galie' N, Humbert M, Vachiery J, et al. ESC/ERS Guidelines for the diagnosis and treatment of pulmonary hypertension. Eur Heart J 2016;37(1):67–119.

4. Vachie'ry J, Adir Y, Barbera JA, et al. Pulmonary hypertension due to left heart diseases. J Am Coll Cardiol 2013;62:D100–8.

5. Simonneau G, Robbins IM, Beghetti M, et al. Updated clinical classification of pulmonary hypertension. J Am Coll Cardiol 2009;54:S43–54.

6. Tampakakis E, Leary PJ, Selby VA, et al. The diastolic pulmonary gradient does not predict survival in patients with pulmonary hypertension due to left heart disease. JACC Heart Fail 2015;3:9–16.

7. Guazzi M, Borlaug BA. Pulmonary hypertension due to left heart disease. Circulation 2012;126:975–90.

8. Rapp AH, Lange RA, Cigarroa JE, et al. Relation of pulmonary arterial diastolic and mean pulmonary arterial wedge pressures in patients with and without pulmonary hypertension. Am J Cardiol 2001;88:823–4.

9. Merlos P, Nunez J, Sanchis J, et al. Echocardiographic estimation of pulmonary arterial systolic pressure in acute heart failure. Prognostic implications. Eur J Intern Med 2013;24(6):562–7.

10. Lam CS, Roger VL, Rodeheffer RJ, et al. Pulmonary hypertension in heart failure with preserved ejection fraction: a community-based study. J Am Coll Cardiol 2009;53:1119–26.

11. Raina A, Abraham WT, Adamson PB, et al. Limitations of right heart catheterization in the diagnosis and risk stratification of patients with pulmonary hypertension related to left heart disease: insights from a wireless pulmonary artery pressure monitoring system. J Heart Lung Transplant 2015;34:438–47.

12. Ghio S, Gavazzi A, Campana C, et al. Independent and additive prognostic value of right ventricular systolic function and pulmonary artery pressure in patients with chronic heart failure. J Am Coll Cardiol 2001;37:183–8.

13. Bursi F, McNallan SM, Redfield MM, et al. Pulmonary pressures and death in heart failure: a community study. J Am Coll Cardiol 2012;59:222–31.

14. Adir Y, Amir O. Pulmonary hypertension associated with left heart disease. Semin Respir Crit Care Med 2013;34:665–80.

15. Lam CS, Borlaug BA, Kane GC, et al. Age-associated increases in pulmonary artery systolic pressure in the general population. Circulation 2009;119(20): 2663–70.

16. Leung CC, Moondra V, Catherwood E, et al. Prevalence and risk factors of pulmonary hypertension in patients with elevated pulmonary venous pressure and preserved ejection fraction. Am J Cardiol 2010;106(2):284–6.

17. Schwartzenberg S, Redfield MM, From AM, et al. Effects of vasodilation in heart failure with preserved or reduced ejection fraction: implications of distinct pathophysiologies on response to therapy. J Am Coll Cardiol 2012;59(5):442–51.

18. Hansdottir S, Groskreutz DJ, Gehlbach BK. WHO's in second? A practical review of World Health Organization group 2 pulmonary hypertension. Chest 2013;144(2):638–50.

19. Gerges M, Gerges C, Pistritto AM, et al. Pulmonary hypertension in heart failure: epidemiology, right ventricular function and survival. Am J Respir Crit Care Med 2015;192:1234–46.

20. Owan TE, Hodge DO, Herges RM, et al. Trends in prevalence and outcome of heart failure with preserved ejection fraction. N Engl J Med 2006; 355(3):251–9.

21. Nkomo VT, Gardin JM, Skelton TN, et al. Burden of valvular heart diseases: a population-based study. Lancet 2006;368:1005–11.

22. Magne J, Pibarot P, Sengupta PP, et al. Pulmonary hypertension in valvular disease. JACC Cardiovasc Imaging 2015;8:83–99.

23. Magne J, Lancellotti P, Pierard LA. Exercise pulmonary hypertension in asymptomatic degenerative mitral regurgitation. Circulation 2010;122: 33–41.

24. Fang JC, DeMarco T, Givertz MM, et al. World Health Organization pulmonary hypertension group 2: pulmonary hypertension due to left heart disease in the adult—a summary statement from the Pulmonary Hypertension Council of the International Society for Heart and Lung Transplantation. J Heart Lung Transplant 2012;31:913–33.

25. Johnson LW, Hapanowicz MB, Buonanno C, et al. Pulmonary hypertension in isolated aortic stenosis. Hemodynamic correlations and follow up. J Thorac Cardiovasc Surg 1988;95(4):603–7.

26. Silver K, Aurigemma G, Krendel S, et al. Pulmonary artery hypertension in severe aortic stenosis: incidence and mechanism. Am Heart J 1992;125: 146–50.

27. Naidoo DP, Mitha AS, Vythilingum S, et al. Pulmonary hypertension in aortic regurgitation: early surgical outcome. Q J Med 1991;80(291):589–95.

28. Lucon A, Oger E, Bedossa M, et al. Prognostic implications of pulmonary hypertension in patients with severe aortic stenosis undergoing transcatheter aortic valve implantation. Circ Cardiovasc Interv 2014;7:240–7.

29. Sinning JM, Hammerstingl C, Chin D, et al. Decrease of pulmonary hypertension impacts on prognosis after transcatheter aortic valve replacement. EuroIntervention 2014;9(9):1042–9.

30. Benza RL, Raina A, Abraham WT, et al. Pulmonary hypertension related to left heart disease: insight from a wireless implantable hemodynamic monitor. J Heart Lung Transplant 2015;34:329–37.

31. Salamon JN, Kelesidis I, Msaouel P, et al. Outcomes in World Health Organization group II pulmonary hypertension: mortality and readmission trends with systolic and preserved ejection fraction-induced pulmonary hypertension. J Card Fail 2014; 20:467–75.

32. Miller WL, Mahoney DW, Enriquez-Sarano M. Quantitative Doppler-echocardiographic imaging and clinical outcomes with left ventricular systolic dysfunction. Independent effect of pulmonary hypertension. Circ Cardiovasc Imaging 2014;7: 330–6.

33. Mohammed SF, Hussain I, AbouEzzeddine OF, et al. Right ventricular function in heart failure with preserved ejection fraction. A community based study. Circulation 2014;130:2310–20.

34. Gerges C, Gerges M, Lang MB, et al. Diastolic pulmonary vascular pressure gradient: a predictor of prognosis in "out of proportion" pulmonary hypertension. Chest 2013;143:758–66.

35. Guazzi M, Gomberg-Maitland M, Arena R. Pulmonary hypertension in heart failure with preserved ejection fraction. J Heart Lung Transplant 2015;34: 273–81.

36. Tedford RJ, Hassoun PM, Mathai SC, et al. Pulmonary capillary wedge pressure augments right ventricular pulsatile loading. Circulation 2012;124: 289–97.

37. Al-Naamani N, Preston IR, Paulus JK, et al. Pulmonary arterial capacitance is an important predictor of mortality in heart failure with a preserved ejection fraction. JACC Heart Fail 2015;3:467–74.

38. Johnson FL. Pathophysiology and etiology of heart failure. Cardiol Clin 2014;32:9–19.

39. Rose-Jones LJ, Rommel JJ, Chang PP. Heart failure with preserved ejection fraction. An ongoing enigma. Cardiol Clin 2014;32:151–61.

40. Pilote L, Huttner I, Marpole D, et al. Stiff left atrial syndrome. Can J Cardiol 1988;4(6):255–7.

41. Mehta S, Charbonneau F, Fitchett DH, et al. The clinical consequences of a stiff left atrium. Am Heart J 1991;122(4 Pt 1):1184–91.

42. Melenovsky V, Hwang S-J, Redfield MM, et al. Left atrial remodeling and function in advanced heart failure with preserved or reduced ejection fraction. Circ Heart Fail 2015;8:295–303.

43. Paulus WJ, Tschope C. A novel paradigm for heart failure with preserved ejection fraction. J Am Coll Cardiol 2013;62:263–71.

44. Kasner M, Westermann D, Lopez B, et al. Diastolic tissue Doppler indexes correlate with the degree of collagen expression and cross-linking in heart failure and normal ejection fraction. J Am Coll Cardiol 2011; 57:977–85.

45. Kottkamp H. Fibrotic atrial cardiomyopathy: a specific disease/syndrome supplying substrates for atrial fibrillation, atrial tachycardia, sinus node disease, and thromboembolic complications. J Cardiovasc Electrophysiol 2012;23:797–9.

46. Hirsh BJ, Copeland-Halperin RS, Halperin JL. Fibrotic atrial cardiomyopathy, atrial fibrillation, and thromboembolism. Mechanistic links and clinical inference. J Am Coll Cardiol 2015;65:2239–51.

47. Khab R, Sheppard R. Fibrosis in heart disease: understanding the role of transforming growth factor-beta in cardiomyopathy, valvular disease and arrhythmia. Immunology 2006;118:10–24.

48. Leask A. Potential therapeutic targets for cardiac fibrosis: TGFB, angiotensin, endothelin, CCN2, and PDGF, partners in fibroblast activation. Circ Res 2010;106:1675–80.

49. Dzeshka MS, Lip GHY, Snezhitskiy V, et al. Cardiac fibrosis in patients with atrial fibrillation: mechanisms and clinical implications. J Am Coll Cardiol 2015;66: 943–59.

50. Hunt JM, Bethea B, Gandjeva A, et al. Pulmonary veins in the normal lung and pulmonary hypertension due to left heart disease. Am J Physiol Lung Cell Mol Physiol 2013;305:L725–36.

51. Huang W, Kingsbury MP, Turner MA, et al. Capillary filtration is reduced in lungs adapted to chronic heart failure: morphological and haemodynamic correlates. Cardiovasc Res 2001;49:207–17.

52. Tsukimoto K, Mathieu-Costello O, Prediletto R, et al. Ultrastructural appearances of pulmonary capillaries at high transmural pressures. J Appl Physiol 1991;71(2):573–82.

53. Palestini P, Calvi C, Conforti E, et al. Composition, biophysical properties, and morphometry of plasma membranes in pulmonary interstitial edema. Am J Physiol Lung Cell Mol Physiol 2002;282:L1382–90.

54. Pietra GG, Capron F, Stewart S, et al. Pathologic assessment of vasculopathies in pulmonary hypertension. J Am Coll Cardiol 2004;43:25S–32S.

55. Berg JT, Breen EC, Fu Z, et al. Alveolar hypoxia increases gene expression of extracellular matrix proteins and platelet-derived growth factor-B in lung parenchyma. Am J Respir Crit Care Med 1998; 158:1920–8.

56. Delgado JF, Conde E, Sa'nchez V, et al. Pulmonary vascular remodeling in pulmonary hypertension

due to chronic heart failure. Eur J Heart Fail 2005;7:
1011–6.

57. Mandegar M, Fung YC, Huang W, et al. Cellular and molecular mechanisms of pulmonary vascular remodeling; role in the development of pulmonary hypertension. Microvasc Res 2004 Sep;68(2):75–103.

58. Rabinovitch M. EVE and beyond, retro and prospective insights. Am J Physiol 1999;277:L5–12.

59. Wagenvoort CA, Mooi WJ. Congestive vasculopathy. In: Wagenvoort CA, Mooi WJ, editors. Biopsy pathology of the pulmonary vasculature. London: Chapman & Hall Medical; 1989. p. 171–98.

60. Klotz S, Deng MC, Hanafy D, et al. Reversible pulmonary hypertension in heart transplant candidates—pretransplant evaluation and outcome after orthotopic heart transplantation. Eur J Heart Fail 2003;5:645–53.

61. Melenovsky V, Al-Hiti H, Kazdova L, et al. Transpulmonary B-type natriuretic peptide uptake and cyclic guanosine monophosphate release in heart failure and pulmonary hypertension: the effects of sildenafil. J Am Coll Cardiol 2009; 54(7):595–600.

62. Cody RJ, Haas GJ, Binkley PF, et al. Plasma endothelin correlates with the extent of pulmonary hypertension in patients with chronic congestive heart failure. Circulation 1992;85:504–9.

63. Hulsmann M, Stanek B, Frey B, et al. Value of cardiopulmonary exercise testing and big endothelin plasma levels to predict short-term prognosis of patients with chronic heart failure. J Am Coll Cardiol 1998;32:1695–700.

64. Kalra PR, Moon JC, Coats AJ. Do results of the ENABLE (Endothelin Antagonist Bosentan for Lowering Cardiac Events in Heart Failure) study spell the end for non-selective endothelin antagonism in heart failure? Int J Cardiol 2002;85:195–7.

65. Guazzi M. Clinical use of phosphodiesterase-5 inhibitors in chronic heart failure. Circ Heart Fail 2008;1:272–80.

66. Forfia PR, Lee M, Tunin RS, et al. Acute phosphodiesterase 5 inhibition mimics hemodynamic effects of B-type natriuretic peptide and potentiates B-type natriuretic peptide effects in failing but not normal canine heart. J Am Coll Cardiol 2007; 49:1079–88.

67. Hamdan R, Mansour H, Nassar P, et al. Prevention of right heart failure after left ventricular assist device implantation by phosphodiesterase 5 inhibitor. Artif Organs 2014;38(11):963–7.

68. Singh RK, Richmond ME, Zuckerman WA, et al. The use of oral sildenafil for management of right ventricular dysfunction after pediatric heart transplantation. Am J Transplant 2014;14(2):453–8.

69. Redfield MM, Chen HH, Borlaug BA, et al. Effect of phosphodiesterase-5 inhibition on exercise capacity and clinical status in heart failure with preserved ejection fraction: a randomized clinical trial. JAMA 2013;309(12):1268–77.

70. Bonderman D, Pretsch I, Steringer-Mascherbauer R, et al. Acute homodynamic effects of riociguat in patients with pulmonary hypertension associated with diastolic heart failure (DILATE-1): a randomized, double blind, placebo-controlled, single-dose study. Chest 2014;146:1274–85.

71. Bonderman D, Ghio S, Felix SB, et al. Riociguat for patients with pulmonary hypertension caused by systolic left ventricular dysfunction. A Phase IIB double-blind, randomized, placebo-controlled, dose-ranging hemodynamic study. Circulation 2013;128:502–11.

72. Rubin LJ. Treatment of pulmonary hypertension caused by left heart failure with pulmonary arterial hypertension-specific therapies. Lessons from the right and LEPHT. Circulation 2013;128: 475–6.

73. Packer M, McMurray J, Massie BM, et al. Clinical effects of endothelin receptor antagonism with bosentan in patients with severe chronic heart failure: results of a pilot study. J Card Fail 2005;11: 12–20.

74. Du L, Sullivan CC, Chu D, et al. Signaling molecules in nonfamilial pulmonary hypertension. N Engl J Med 2003;348(6):500–9.

75. Olson TP, Snyder EM, Frantz RP, et al. Repeat length polymorphism of the serotonin transporter gene influences pulmonary artery pressure in heart failure. Am Heart J 2007;153(3):426–32.

76. Haddad F, Hunt SA, Rosenthal DN, et al. Right ventricular function in cardiovascular disease, part I: anatomy, physiology, aging, and functional assessment of the right ventricle. Circulation 2008;117: 1436–48.

77. Guihaire J, Noly PE, Schrepfer S, et al. Advancing knowledge of right ventricular pathophysiology in chronic pressure overload: insights from experimental studies. Arch Cardiovasc Dis 2015;108(10): 519–29.

78. Haddad F, Doyle R, Murphy DJ, et al. Right ventricular function in cardiovascular disease, part II: pathophysiology, clinical importance, and management of right ventricular failure. Circulation 2008;117: 1717–31.

79. Melenovsky V, Hwang SJ, Lin G, et al. Right heart dysfunction in heart failure with preserved ejection fraction. Eur Heart J 2014;35:3452–62.

80. Morrison D, Goldman S, Wright AL, et al. The effect of pulmonary hypertension on systolic function of the right ventricle. Chest 1983;84:250–7.

81. Rouleau JL, Kapuku G, Pelletier S, et al. Cardioprotective effects of ramipril and losartan in right ventricular pressure overload in the rabbit: importance of kinins and influence of angiotensin II type 1

receptor signaling pathway. Circulation 2001;104: 939–44.

82. Borgdorff MA, Dickinson MG, Berger RM, et al. Right ventricular failure due to chronic pressure load: what have we learned in animal models since the NIH working group statement? Heart Fail Rev 2015;20:475–91.

83. Potus F, Ruffenach G, Dahou A, et al. Downregulation of miR-126 contributes to the failing right ventricle in pulmonary arterial hypertension. Circulation 2015;132(10):932–43.

84. Dromparis P, Michelakis ED. Mitochondria in vascular health and disease. Annu Rev Physiol 2013;75:95–126.

85. Talati M, Hemnes A. Fatty acid metabolism in pulmonary arterial hypertension: role in right ventricular dysfunction and hypertrophy. Pulm Circ 2015;5(2): 269–78.

86. Thompson JT, Rackley MS, O'Brien TX. Upregulation of the cardiac homeobox gene Nkx2-5 (CSX) in feline right ventricular pressure overload. Am J Physiol 1998;274:H1569–73.

87. Jensen BC, O'Connell TD, Simpson PC. Alpha-1-adrenergic receptors in heart failure: the adaptive

arm of the cardiac response to chronic catecholamine stimulation. J Cardiovasc Pharmacol 2014; 63(4):291–301.

88. Hoper MM, Bogaard HJ, Condliffe R, et al. Definitions and diagnosis of pulmonary hypertension. J Am Coll Cardiol 2013;62:D42–50.

89. Costard-Jackle A, Fowler MB. Influence of preoperative pulmonary artery pressure on mortality after heart transplantation: testing of potential reversibility of pulmonary hypertension with nitroprusside is useful in defining a high risk group. J Am Coll Cardiol 1992;19:48–54.

90. Fox BD, Shimony A, Langleben D, et al. High prevalence of occult left heart disease in scleroderma-pulmonary hypertension. Eur Respir J 2013;42: 1083–91.

91. Andersen MF, Olson TP, Melenovsky V, et al. Differential hemodynamic effects of exercise and volume expansion in people with and without heart failure. Circ Heart Fail 2015;8(1):41–8.

92. Herve P, Lau EM, Sibon O, et al. Criteria for diagnosis of exercise pulmonary hypertension. Eur Respir J 2015;46(3):728–37.

Group III Pulmonary Hypertension
Pulmonary Hypertension Associated with Lung Disease: Epidemiology, Pathophysiology, and Treatments

James R. Klinger, MD

KEYWORDS

- Pulmonary hypertension • Chronic obstructive pulmonary disease • Interstitial lung disease
- Obstructive sleep apnea • Endothelin receptor antagonist • Phosphodiesterase inhibitor
- Prostacyclin • Soluble guanylate cyclase stimulator

KEY POINTS

- Pulmonary hypertension occurs frequently in most chronic lung diseases, but is usually moderate with mean pulmonary artery pressure in the range of 20 to 30 mm Hg.
- The presence of even moderate pulmonary hypertension in chronic lung disease is associated with increased morbidity and mortality.
- The cause of pulmonary hypertension in chronic lung disease is multifactorial and includes loss of peripheral pulmonary vessels, chronic or recurrent hypoxia, and altered expression of vascular and inflammatory mediators.
- Management should be directed at treating the underlying lung disease because currently available medications for the treatment of pulmonary arterial hypertension have not been found to be effective for the treatment of pulmonary hypertension associated with chronic lung disease.
- Patients with severe pulmonary hypertension and mild to moderate lung disease may deserve consideration for enrollment in clinical trials or referral to centers experienced in the management of pulmonary arterial hypertension.

INTRODUCTION

Increased pulmonary arterial pressure (PAP) is a common feature of many chronic lung diseases and chronic lung disease is the second most common cause of pulmonary hypertension (PH).[1] PH caused by chronic lung disease is referred to as group 3 PH in the most recent classification scheme presented by the World Health Organization (WHO) meetings on PH (see Oudiz RJ: Classification of Pulmonary Hypertension, in this issue). Screening studies suggest that approximately a quarter of all patients with increased PAP have WHO group 3 PH.[1] The most common lung diseases in WHO group 3 PH are chronic obstructive pulmonary disease (COPD), interstitial lung disease (ILD), and obstructive sleep apnea (OSA). PH associated with pulmonary sarcoidosis

Conflicts of Interest: Dr J.R. Klinger receives grant support from the National Heart, Lung, and Blood Institute (RO1 HL 123965) and the following pharmaceutical companies: Bayer, Gilead, Lung Biotechnology, United Therapeutics.
Division of Pulmonary, Sleep and Critical Care Medicine, Alpert Medical School of Brown University, Rhode Island Hospital, Ambulatory Patient Center, Room 701, 593 Eddy Street, Providence, RI 02903, USA
E-mail address: james_klinger@brown.edu

Cardiol Clin 34 (2016) 413–433
http://dx.doi.org/10.1016/j.ccl.2016.04.003
0733-8651/16/$ – see front matter © 2016 Elsevier Inc. All rights reserved.

and Langerhans histiocytosis X are classified as WHO group 5 PH (see Tannenbaum SK, Gomberg-Maitland M: Group 5 Pulmonary Hypertension: The Orphan's Orphan Disease, in this issue). The presence of PH in chronic lung disease is strongly associated with decreased survival, decreased functional capacity, and increased complications. However, it is unclear whether PH is the cause of worse outcome in these patients or simply a marker of more advanced lung disease.

Although treatment of the underlying lung condition remains the primary approach to managing PH associated with chronic lung disease, this is often easier said than done. PH often occurs in advanced lung diseases that are usually irreversible. When little else remains to be done for a patient's lung disease, health care providers often look to other associated conditions that might be addressed in order to improve the outcome of the patient. The large number of drugs that have been developed and approved for WHO group 1 pulmonary arterial hypertension (PAH) over the last 20 years has made it increasingly difficult to resist the temptation of using these medications to treat PH associated with chronic lung disease. Furthermore, the strong negative correlation between pulmonary artery (PA) pressure and survival in most lung diseases makes it seem reasonable that any success at treating PH in these patients should improve their outcomes. However, findings from a limited number of studies that have attempted to address this issue do not suggest that this is the case.

Two important questions need to be considered when treating PH associated with chronic lung disease: (1) are currently available medications able to improve pulmonary vascular resistance (PVR) in chronic lung disease, and (2) does improving pulmonary hemodynamics in chronic lung disease improve patient outcome? The latter question is particularly important because, unlike patients with idiopathic PAH, those with PH associated with lung disease may be more limited by impairments in ventilation than by cardiac output (CO).

This article reviews the pathophysiology of PH associated with lung disease and summarizes the clinical data that have been generated. Although there are currently no medical therapies that are approved or even recommended for the treatment of PH associated with chronic lung disease, the benefits and limitations of currently available therapies are discussed along with an approach to selecting patients and deciding under what conditions treatment of PH should be attempted.

EPIDEMIOLOGY

The pulmonary circulation is a low-pressure system that normally maintains a small pressure gradient between the pulmonary arterial and pulmonary venous circulations. In healthy adults, mean PAP (mPAP) is 14.0 ± 3.3 mm Hg[2,3] and right ventricular systolic pressures (RVSPs) are in the range of 24 to 30 mm Hg.[4] Therefore, mPAP of 21 mm Hg, which would result in an RVSP of 35 to 40 mm Hg, is about 2 standard deviations greater than the mean and would be considered to be abnormal. As a result, mPAP of 20 mm Hg and/or RVSP of 35 mm Hg have been used as cutoff values to define PH in many studies, particularly those examining PH in lung disease. However, PAP increases slowly with age and mPAP in patients with Group 1 PAH is well beyond 2 standard deviations from the mean, averaging 50 to 55 mm Hg in most registries.[4–7] As a result, the most widely accepted definition of PH is a mPAP greater than or equal to 25 mm Hg.[2]

In contrast with the near-systemic PAPs seen in patients with PAH, the increase in PAP in patients with chronic lung disease tends to be mild to moderate, with most studies reporting mPAP in the range of 25 to 35 mm Hg. Increase of mPAP to levels normally seen in PAH is rare. Most studies report that only about 3% to 4% of patients with chronic lung disease have mPAP greater than 40 mm Hg. This finding shows one of the marked differences between group 1 PAH and group 3 PH and points to important differences in the underlying pathophysiology and pulmonary vascular remodeling.

Prevalence of Pulmonary Hypertension in Patients with Chronic Obstructive Pulmonary Disease

The true incidence of PH in COPD has been difficult to establish, but most studies reported PH in 30% to 70% of patients.[8–10] This broad range in prevalence rates is attributable to several factors, including differences in the severity of COPD in the population studied, minor differences in the definition used for PH, and differences in the techniques used to assess PAP. Studies using transthoracic echocardiography (TTE) to measure PAP and defining PH as systolic PAP (sPAP) greater than 40 mm Hg report a prevalence of about 35% to 50%. However, TTE has considerable limitations in accurately measuring PAP in patients with chronic lung disease. In one often-cited study the correlation between sPAP estimated by TTE and measured by right heart catheterization (RHC) in patients with advanced lung disease was good ($r = 0.69$; $P<.0001$), but varied by more than 10 mm Hg in slightly more than half (52%) of the patients studied.[11] In that study, 48% of patients were incorrectly classified by TTE as having PH.

Data are limited regarding pulmonary hemodynamics measured by RHC in patients with mild to moderate COPD because it is difficult to justify an invasive procedure as a screening tool in studies of mildly symptomatic patients. However, several studies have reported RHC data in patients with advanced COPD. For example, a retrospective review of 156 patients with COPD referred for lung transplant evaluation found that the mPAP was 25 ± 6 mm Hg with a PVR index (PVRi) of 4.4 Wood units/m².[12] In the same study, pulmonary hemodynamics in 77 patients with idiopathic pulmonary fibrosis (IPF) were similar with mPAP 27 ± 12 mm[12] Hg and PVRi 6.2 ± 5.4 mm Hg/L/min/m². By comparison, mPAP in 50 patients with PAH was 58 ± 21 mm Hg and PVRi was 24 ± 11.6 mm Hg/L/min/m².[12] A later retrospective study examined 215 patients with severe COPD who underwent RHC as part of an evaluation for lung transplant or lung volume reduction surgery.[13] PH defined as mPAP greater than 25 mm Hg was found in 50.2% of patients. However, mPAP again was only slightly increased (26.9 mm Hg). Only about 10% had mPAP greater than 35 mm Hg and less than 4% had mPAP greater than 45 mm Hg. The prevalence of PH in 120 patients with COPD who underwent RHC in the National Emphysema Treatment Trial (NETT) was reported to be as high as 91%.[14] However, mPAP was no different than what was reported in other trials (26.3 ± 5.2 mm Hg) and only 5% of patients had mPAP greater than 35 mm Hg. The reason for the much higher prevalence of PH in the NETT study is that PH was defined as mPAP greater than 20 mm Hg instead of greater than 25 mm Hg. Perhaps the best estimates of PH prevalence in severe COPD comes from a retrospective review of 4930 patients from the Organ Procurement and Tissue Network (OPTN) database for all patients with COPD listed for transplant between 1997 and 2006.[15] PH defined as mPAP greater than or equal to 25 mm Hg was present in 2346 (47.6%), although 847 patients (17.2%) had PA occlusion pressure (PAOP) greater than or equal to 15 mm Hg (**Fig. 1**). Again, only a small minority (4%) had mPAP greater than 35 mm Hg.

The findings from these studies are consistent and show that most patients with advanced COPD have mPAP between 20 and 30 mm Hg. Although this range of pressure is clearly abnormal to the extent that about half of the patients have PH as defined by modern criteria, very few

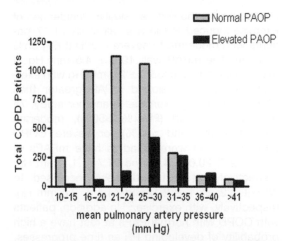

Fig. 1. PAPs with normal and increased PAOP in 4930 patients with a primary diagnosis of COPD in the OPTN database between 1997 and 2006. (*From* Cuttica MJ, Kalhan R, Shlobin OA, et al. Categorization and impact of pulmonary hypertension in patients with advanced COPD. Respir Med 2010;104(12):1880; with permission.)

patients have increases of mPAP that approach those of the average patient with PAH.

In general, the prevalence of PH seems to be lower in patients with less severe COPD. Several small studies of patients with COPD with forced expiratory volume in 1 second (FEV₁) approximately 40% of predicted report prevalence rates for PH from 35% to 43% when defined as mPAP greater than 20 mm Hg.[16,17] In one study, mPAP was greater than 26 mm Hg in just 20% of patients.[18] Studies using TTE to estimate PA systolic pressure have also found prevalence rates of about 50% for PH in moderate COPD. In one study,[19] sPAP was assessed by TTE in 73 consecutive patients with COPD who attended a hospital outpatient clinic. Transtricuspid pressure gradient (TTPG; the difference between RVSP and right atrial pressure) could be calculated in 77% of patients and PH, defined as TTPG greater than or equal to 30 mm Hg, was found in 55%. In a retrospective review, our group reported that 2 out of 3 patients with COPD (105 out of 159) had a sufficient TTPG to measure sPAP and that PH, defined as sPAP greater than or equal to 36 mm Hg, was present in 60%.[20]

The prevalence of exercise-induced PH in COPD is even higher. In a study by Oswald-Mammosser and colleagues,[21] mPAP was greater than 20 mm Hg in only 31 of 151 patients with moderate COPD (percentage of FEV₁ [FEV₁%], 38% ± 12% predicted), but increased to greater than or equal to 30 mm Hg with exercise (up to 40 W) in 99 patients (66%). Christensen and colleagues[22] showed a similar incidence of exercise-induced PH in a small study of 17 patients with moderate to severe COPD (FEV_1 35% ± 10%). The mPAP was 19.9 ± 4.5 mm Hg at rest, but increased to 35.0 ± 2.2 mm Hg with exercise and 65% developed mPAP greater than 30 mm Hg during exercise. In another study, 75 patients with mild (FEV_1% >50%), moderate (FEV_1% <50% and >35%), or severe COPD (FEV_1% ≤35%) were found to have mPAPs of 21.5 ± 2.7, 20.0 ± 4.2, and 21.7 ± 1.1 mm Hg, respectively, at rest and these increased to 32.7 ± 3.2, 38.1 ± 2.1, and 44.4 ± 2.0 mm Hg, respectively, with exercise.[23] In addition, patients with COPD with normal PAPs at rest have a high probability of developing PH as time progresses. In an often-cited study, Kessler and colleagues[24] measured pulmonary hemodynamics by RHC in a group of 131 patients with moderate COPD (FEV_1%, 34.6% ± 15.7%) and mPAP less than 20 mm Hg and followed them for a mean interval of 6.8 ± 2.9 years. Twenty-five percent of patients developed PH, defined as mPAP greater than 20 mm Hg during the study period, and the average rate of increase in mPAP was 0.4 mm Hg/y. Patients who developed PH had higher mPAPs at rest and during exercise at the beginning of the study.

Prevalence of Pulmonary Hypertension in Patients with Interstitial Lung Disease

The prevalence and severity of PH in ILD is similar to those of COPD and the same obstacles to obtaining accurate prevalence rates pertain. As with COPD, estimation of PAPs by TTE is limited. In the study by Arcosay and colleagues[11] cited earlier the sensitivity, specificity, and positive and negative predictive values of TTE to detect a sPAP greater than 45 mm Hg were 85%, 17%, 60%, and 44%, respectively. Prevalence rates of PH in patients with advanced ILD have been reported between 32% and 84%.[25–29] In one of the largest studies,[26] 46% of 2525 patients with ILD listed for lung transplant with the United Network for Organ Sharing and the Organ Procurement and Transplant Network registry had PH defined as mPAP greater than 25 mm Hg by RHC. Only 9% had severe PH defined as mPAP greater than 40 mm Hg.

Prevalence of Pulmonary Hypertension in Sleep Disordered Breathing

Determining the prevalence and severity of PH in patients with sleep disordered breathing (SDB) is complicated by the common occurrence of comorbidities that can contribute to increased PAP. Most forms of SDB, such as OSA and obesity hypoventilation syndrome (OHS), occur more frequently in patients with obesity. These patients often have concomitant hypertensive cardiovascular disease with impairments in left ventricular function that result in pulmonary venous hypertension. Approximately 10% to 15% of patients with OSA also have COPD and PH occurs more commonly in this group. In addition, data are accruing to suggest that obesity and its associated metabolic syndrome of insulin resistance, endothelial dysfunction, and increased oxidative stress is a risk factor for the development of PH.[30,31]

As with other chronic lung disease, prevalence rates of PH in SDB vary greatly. The lack of large-scale studies with clearly defined patient populations makes it difficult to determine the true prevalence rate, but most studies suggest that about 20% to 30% of patients with OSA have some degree of PH. In a recent review, Ismail and colleagues[32] cited 8 studies that reported prevalence rates of PH in OSA from 17% to 70%. However, all but 1 of these studies defined PH as mPAP greater than 20 mm Hg as opposed to greater than 25 mm Hg. In the 1 study that reported a prevalence of 70%,[33] most patients had pulmonary capillary wedge pressures greater than 15 mm Hg. When these patients were excluded, the prevalence rate for PH decreased to 22%. Despite differences in prevalence rates, all 8 studies consistently reported mild increases in PAP, with mPAP averaging less than 30 mm Hg. In one of the largest studies to date, the prevalence rate of PH in 220 patients with SDB was 17% and the mPAP was 26 ± 6 mm Hg.[34] The other consistent finding in most studies was that PH correlated with the severity of obesity, daytime hypoxia and hypercapnia, obstructive airway disease, and nocturnal oxygen desaturation. PH seems to be more common and more severe in OHS than in OSA, with prevalence rates of 58% and 88% reported in 2 different studies.[35,36] OSA also occurs commonly in patients with PAH, making it difficult to determine which disease is causing which.

Severe Pulmonary Hypertension in Chronic Lung Disease

Although PH associated with chronic lung disease tends to be moderate, some patients develop PAP that is as severe as that seen in WHO group 1 PAH. For these patients it becomes difficult to determine whether they represent the extreme end of the spectrum of PH in lung disease or whether they have developed PAH in addition to their lung disease. These patients are often referred to as having PH that is out of proportion to their underlying lung disease, but this label can be misleading because there are no generally accepted criteria for what degree of PAP increase is appropriate for the severity of lung disease. Thus, it may be better to refer to this type of PH as simply severe PH, usually indicating mPAP greater than 35 to 40 mm Hg. This cutoff level seems to be important, because it occurs rarely even in patients with advanced lung disease and may signify the presence of another disease process or abnormal pulmonary vascular response.

Several studies have attempted to better define the clinical phenotype of patients with chronic lung disease who have severe PH. In a retrospective review of 998 patients with COPD, from a single institution, who underwent RHC, only 27 (2.7%) had severe PH defined as mPAP greater than 40 mm Hg.[37] In 16 of these 27, other comorbid conditions, including connective tissue disease, anorexigen use, portal hypertension, history of pulmonary embolism, left heart disease, and restrictive lung disease, were identified that could have contributed to the development of PH. In the other 11, there was no apparent cause of the severe PH other than COPD. These patients were all men aged 54 to 77 years. Most were heavy smokers with moderate to severe airway obstruction and all were hypoxemic. The carbon monoxide diffusion in the lung (DLco), measured in 9 patients, was extremely low (median 4.6 mL/min/mm Hg) and high-resolution computed tomography consistently showed emphysema. Right-to-left shunting measured in 8 patients was abnormally high, with a median of 19% shunt. Despite severe PH and severely reduced DLco (4.6) and Pao$_2$ (46 mm Hg), these patients had modest airways disease, with a median FEV$_1$ of 50% predicted (IQR (interquartile range) 45%–56%) and were mildly hypocapnic (Paco$_2$ 32 mm Hg). Although severe PH was uncommon, the prevalence rate in this study (1.1%) is similar to the prevalence of PAH in other diseases, such as human immunodeficiency virus and portal hypertension (0.5% and 2.0%, respectively), and raises the question of whether or not COPD is a risk factor for developing PAH. At the same time, patients with PAH often have COPD. In the ASPIRE registry, 1737 consecutive, incident, treatment-naive patients were referred for evaluation of suspected PH.[38] After extensive evaluation including RHC, 101 patients were diagnosed with PH associated with COPD and 32 with PH associated with ILD. Fifty-nine of the 101 patients with COPD had mPAP greater than 40 mm Hg. Compared with the other 42 patients, those with severe PH had lower DLco, but less severe airflow obstruction. In a retrospective review of 215 patients with COPD, Thabut and colleagues[13] reported mPAP greater than 35 mm Hg in 13.5% and mPAP greater than 50 mm Hg in only 3%. A subgroup of patients with severe PH were characterized by lower oxygen levels and higher FEV$_1$. Correlation between Pao$_2$ and PAP was good (mean $r = -0.55$; $P = .0001$), whereas correlation with FEV$_1$ was only $r = -0.17$ ($P<.05$) (**Fig. 2**). Severe PH has also been reported in patients with SDB, particularly in patients with OHS. In one early study of PH in OHS, the prevalence of severe PH, defined as mPAP greater than 40 mm Hg, was 31%.[36]

Patients with severe PH associated with chronic lung disease are characterized by lower oxygenation, lower DLco, and often less severe reductions in FEV$_1$.

Effect of Pulmonary Hypertension on Prognosis

PH has been found to be a poor prognostic indicator in chronic lung diseases including COPD, ILD, and OSA (**Fig. 3**). Numerous studies have shown that PH negatively affects survival in COPD.[39] Furthermore, patients with severe PH have worse survival than patients with moderate PH[38,40] (**Fig. 4**). A retrospective review at our institution

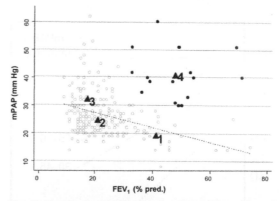

Fig. 2. Correlation between the FEV$_1$ (%pred.) and mPAP in patients with COPD. The correlation is modest. Patients with severely reduced FEV$_1$% have a wide range of mPAP from near normal to severely increased and patients with low mPAP have a wide range of FEV$_1$%. Patients are grouped into 4 categories: (1) mild PH and mild COPD, (2) mild PH and severe COPD, (3) severe PH and severe COPD, and (4) severe PH and mild COPD. The fourth group, although only a small minority, may be most likely to benefit from treatment of PH. (*From* Thabut G, Dauriat G, Stern JB, et al. Pulmonary hemodynamics in advanced COPD candidates for lung volume reduction surgery or lung transplantation. Chest 2005;127(5):1535; with permission.)

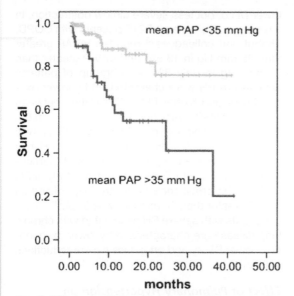

Fig. 3. Effect of mPAP on survival in 176 consecutive patients with various pulmonary diseases, most of which were COPD (n = 45) and ILD (n = 55). (*From* Leuchte HH, Baumgartner RA, Nounou ME, et al. Brain natriuretic peptide is a prognostic parameter in chronic lung disease. Am J Respir Crit Care Med 2006;173(7):748; with permission.)

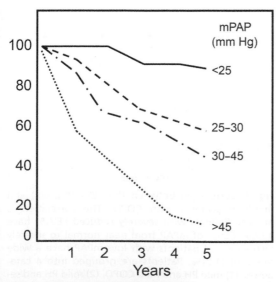

Fig. 4. Effect of mPAP on survival in patients with COPD according to severity of mPAP increase. Note the marked negative effect on survival as PH becomes more severe. (*Adapted from* Naeije R, MacNee W. Pulmonary circulation. In: Calverley P, MacNee W, Pride P, editors. Chronic obstructive pulmonary disease. 2nd edition. London: Arnold Health Sciences; 2003. p. 239; with permission.)

found that 16 of 23 patients (70%) with PH, defined as RVSP greater than 45 mm Hg on echocardiography during hospital admission for COPD exacerbation, died during a 1-year follow-up period compared with 5 of 20 patients (25%) without PH (P = .0058).[41] No other variables measured, including age, best or worst Pao_2, $Paco_2$, or pH, were associated with mortality.

Increased PAP has also been shown to correlate with morbidity, including increased hospital admission rate. In a study by Kessler and colleagues,[42] the rate of hospitalization in patients with COPD with PH was twice that of those without it and PAP and Pco_2 were the only independent predictors of hospitalization. In most studies that find a correlation between PAP and adverse outcome, other independent predictors have usually included oxygenation and DLco.

Most studies suggest that FEV_1 correlates inversely with PAP in COPD.[13,20] PH is more common in patients with severe airways disease, but the correlation between PAP and airway disease as assessed by pulmonary function tests (PFTs) does not seem to be as strong (see **Fig. 2**). These findings suggest that the increase in PAP responsible for the adverse effect on outcome is associated with decreased gas exchange and may be caused by a loss of vessels at the alveolar/capillary level.

The presence of PH also has a negative impact on morbidity and mortality associated with ILD. In a study that divided patients into 3 groups based on echocardiographic assessment of RVSP, the Kaplan-Meier median survival rates for patients with RVSP less than 35 mm Hg (14 patients), 36 to 50 mm Hg (47 patients), and greater than 50 mm Hg (27 patients) were 4.8 years, 4.1 years, and 0.7 years, respectively (P = .009).[43] In another study that reported 5-year survival in 61 patients with IPF who had pulmonary hemodynamics measured by RHC, 23 of 37 patients (62.2%) with mPAP less than 17 mm Hg survived for 5 years, whereas only 4 of 24 patients (16.7%) with mPAP greater than 17 mm Hg survived (P<.001).[44] The 5-year mortality was nearly 4-fold greater in patients with PH, although mPAP in these patients was only 21 ± 4 mm Hg. The presence of PH in ILD is also associated with decreased functional capacity and quality of life.[45,46]

PH is associated with increased morbidity and mortality in chronic lung disease and the adverse effect on outcome correlates with the severity of PH.

PATHOPHYSIOLOGY

As discussed earlier, the pulmonary circulation is a low-pressure system with little basal vascular tone and most of the resistance to flow is caused by the normal narrowing and branching of the pulmonary vascular bed. When CO increases, such as during vigorous exercise, the increase in blood flow is accommodated by dilatation of perfused vessels and recruitment of underperfused vessels. As a result, CO can increase 3-fold to 4-fold during heavy exercise with little increase in PAP. The greater increase in CO than in PAP means that, in the healthy lung, PVR (defined as PAP/CO) decreases during exercise. Pathology studies and pulmonary angiography studies have shown that patients with chronic lung disease such as COPD have fewer peripheral pulmonary blood vessels.[10] This loss of blood vessels reduces the number that can be recruited when CO increases and is likely one of the reasons why exercise-induced PH is so commonly seen in patients with COPD and ILD.[21–24]

Most lung diseases result in chronic or intermittent periods of hypoxia. Unlike the microcirculation of the systemic vascular bed, which dilates in response to hypoxia, pulmonary vascular tone increases in response to decreased oxygen tension. Hypoxic pulmonary vasoconstriction (HPVC) occurs in response to both alveolar hypoxia and pulmonary arterial hypoxemia and is enhanced by hypercapnia or academia.[47,48] Note that both can be present despite fairly normal systemic oxygenation saturation, because of a compensatory mechanism to maintain systemic arterial oxygenation. For example, HPVC works to maintain normal arterial O_2 tension by diverting pulmonary blood flow away from areas of alveolar hypoxia. When large areas of the lung have impaired ventilation, HPVC can still correct systemic O_2 saturation to near normal, but this occurs at the expense of increased pulmonary vascular tone. Although HPVC is usually reversible with supplemental oxygen, sustained or repeated exposure to hypoxia results in increased muscularization of the pulmonary vascular bed and remodeling of the distal pulmonary circulation that is only partially reversed on correction of hypoxia. The relationship between the severity of hypoxia and the severity of PAP increase is a consistent finding in PH associated with chronic lung disease. Several studies have shown that Pao_2 as well as $DLco$ correlate inversely with measures of PAP.[10,14,20,37]

Alveolar hypoxia need not be continuous to produce PH. Right ventricular hypertrophy (RVH) develops with as little as 2 hours a day of hypoxia and abnormal pulmonary hemodynamics have been reported in patients with nocturnal hypoxia secondary to OSA.[49] Furthermore, there is considerable individual variation in the degree of HPVC that occurs in response to acute hypoxia[50] and this variability has also been observed in patients

with COPD and OSA.[51,52] This finding means that some patients show a marked increase in PAP and PVR during acute hypoxia and are likely predisposed to developing more pulmonary vascular remodeling when exposed to persistent or recurrent alveolar hypoxia (**Fig. 5**). The pulmonary vascular response to hypoxia may be genetically predetermined. In a study of 67 hypoxemic patients with COPD, 21 patients who carried the LL 5HTT (serotonin transporter) gene polymorphism, which is associated with higher levels of 5HTT, had mPAPs of 34 ± 13 mm Hg compared with 23 ± 5 mm Hg in 34 LS patients ($P<.002$) and 22 ± 4 mm Hg in 12 SS patients ($P<.005$).[53] The degree of airway obstruction and hypoxemia were similar in all 3 groups.

The PVR may also be affected by changes in lung volume. In general, extra-alveolar vessels are mildly distended by the negative pressure of the interstitium and dilate as the lung is inflated, whereas intra-alveolar vessels are compressed between alveoli during inflation and increase resistance. These forces act in opposite directions and offset each other most at functional residual capacity (FRC).[54] As such, changes in lung volume more than or less than FRC usually increase PVR.

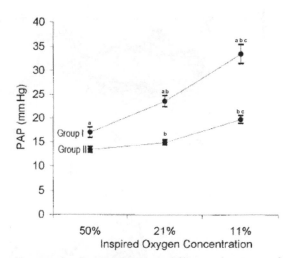

Fig. 5. Change in mPAP at different fractions of inspired oxygen in patients with obstructive sleep apnea with (group 1) and without (group 2) PH (defined as mPAP >20 mm Hg while breathing room air at rest). The hypoxic pressor response measured as the difference in PAP between 50% and 11% oxygen breathing was greater in group I than in group II patients. [a] $P<.05$ versus group II, [b] $P<.05$ versus 50% oxygen breathing, [c] $P<.05$ versus 21% oxygen breathing. (*From* Sajkov D, Wang T, Saunders NA, et al. Daytime pulmonary hemodynamics in patients with obstructive sleep apnea without lung disease. Am J Respir Crit Care Med 1999;159(5 Pt 1):1522; with permission.)

It may not be surprising that PH is common in chronic lung diseases like COPD and ILD that affect the lung diffusely enough to alter gas exchange and lung volume. However, the question arises as to whether PH associated with chronic lung disease is an unavoidable consequence of the underlying damage that is done to the lung or whether the chronic lung diseases are capable of inciting a pulmonary vascular disease that is separate from or out of proportion to the underlying lung injury. Several lines of evidence suggest that the latter may be correct. First, neither the prevalence nor the severity of PH that is seen in patients with chronic lung disease correlate well with measures of pulmonary function.[27] Although most studies have found an inverse correlation between low DLco and PAP in IPF,[27] it is not clear whether the reduction in DLco in these patients contributes to the development of PH or the development of PH results in a decrease in DLco. The second line of evidence is that histopathologic examination of patients with IPF shows evidence of vascular remodeling in areas of normal lung. In one study[55] of lungs obtained from patients with IPF who were transplanted, 65% of patients had evidence of pulmonary arterial thickening and occlusion of small

pulmonary veins and venules in areas of preserved lung architecture (**Fig. 6**). In addition, many abnormalities in expression of inflammatory mediators and growth factors that have been implicated in the pathogenesis of PAH are present in PH associated with lung disease. For example, pulmonary expression of the endothelium-derived vasoconstrictor endothelin-1 (ET-1) is increased in patients with PAH and circulating levels correlate with disease severity.[56,57] Similarly, plasma ET-I levels have also been shown to be higher in patients with emphysema and ILD and to correlate with PAP at rest and during exercise.[58] Increased expression of endothelin-converting enzyme has been observed in type II pneumocytes of patients with IPF.[59] Furthermore, genetic overexpression of ET-1 causes pulmonary fibrosis in mice,[60] raising the question of whether ET-1 contributes to the pathogenesis of ILD and the PH that develops in many patients with this disease. Similarly, overexpression of interleukin-6 (IL-6) has been implicated in the pathogenesis of PAH[61] and IL-6 levels are increased in the bronchoalveolar lavage fluid of patients with IPF.[62] Decreased bioavailability of nitric oxide (NO) in the pulmonary circulation is also thought to play a key role in the

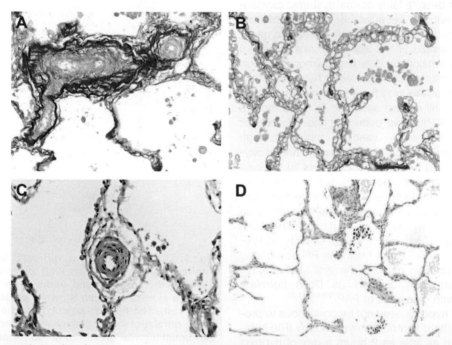

Fig. 6. Lung sections taken from a patient with PH and pulmonary fibrosis. Note that C shows pulmonary vascular remodeling with medial hyperplasia in a vessel distant from areas of fibrosis. (A) Elastic stain highlights the occlusion of a preseptal vein by fibrous tissue. (B) alveolar capillary multiplication. (C) muscularization of pulmonary arteriole. (D) Iron deposition in alveolar macrophages. (Sections were stained with hematoxylin and eosin, elastic stain for vessel identification, and Perls' method for iron). (From Colombat M, Mal H, Groussard O, et al. Pulmonary vascular lesions in end-stage idiopathic pulmonary fibrosis: Histopathologic study on lung explant specimens and correlations with pulmonary hemodynamics. Hum Pathol 2007;38(1):63; with permission.)

development of pulmonary vascular disease,[63] and expression of endothelial NO synthase, the key enzyme responsible for NO synthesis in the pulmonary vasculature, is decreased in the lungs of cigarette smokers (**Fig. 7**).[64] Recent studies suggest that impaired NO synthesis caused by tobacco smoke causes apoptosis of pulmonary vascular endothelial cells and leads to the development of PH and emphysema.[65] Several other mediators that are abnormally expressed in PAH have also been found to be dysregulated in chronic lung diseases, including C-reactive protein, tumor necrosis factor-alpha, transforming growth factor-beta, and vascular endothelial growth factor.[65–68] These findings raise the possibility that chronic lung diseases produce an environment that is prone to the induction of a pulmonary vascular disease that is similar to PAH. If so, medications that have been found to be effective for PAH should be effective for treating PH in chronic lung disease or even the underlying lung disease. However, as reviewed later, most studies conducted thus far have not found this to be the case.

Numerous factors likely contribute to the increase of PVR in chronic lung disease, but the most important seem to be the loss and remodeling of distal prealveolar pulmonary arterioles; increased vascular tone and muscularization of distal, normally nonmuscularized, vessels caused by chronic or recurrent hypoxia; and abnormal expression of a variety of vascular and inflammatory mediators, many of which have been found to be similarly dysregulated in PAH.

TREATMENT OF PULMONARY HYPERTENSION ASSOCIATED WITH LUNG DISEASE
Treatment of Pulmonary Hypertension Associated with Chronic Obstructive Pulmonary Disease

Studies designed to reduce PAP in COPD began in the 1970s with studies examining the efficacy of supplemental oxygen. One of the primary hypotheses was that oxygen would relieve hypoxic pulmonary vasoconstriction and reduce PAP, thereby unloading the right ventricle and improving exercise capacity. Two large, multicenter studies were conducted to determine the effects of long-term oxygen therapy (LTo_2) on pulmonary hemodynamics, patient function, and survival. The Medical Research Council Working Party studied 87 patients in the United Kingdom with chronic bronchitis, emphysema, and hypoxemia.[69] Patients were randomly assigned to receive oxygen for 15 hours a day or no oxygen and were followed for up to 5 years. After 500 days, patients receiving LTo_2 had half the mortality of those not receiving LTo_2 (12% vs 29%). mPAP and PVR remained steady in patients receiving LTo_2 and increased in control subjects, but the improvement in survival did not correlate with change in pulmonary hemodynamics measured during the first year of therapy. In North America, the Nocturnal Oxygen Therapy Trial studied 203 hypoxic patients with COPD and randomized them to receive either nocturnal (average 12 h/d) or continuous (average 17.7 h/d) LTo_2.[70] Mortalities in the nocturnal

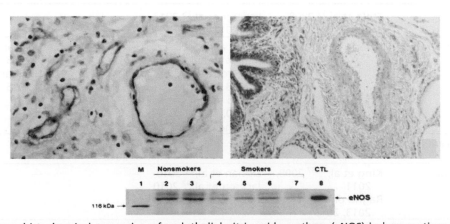

Fig. 7. Immunohistochemical expression of endothelial nitric oxide synthase (eNOS) in lung sections of smokers and nonsmokers. (*Left*) Intense staining of endothelial cells for eNOS in a small PA and capillaries (original magnification ×400). (*Right*) eNOS immunoreactivity in a smoker, showing marked staining in bronchial epithelium and bronchial vessels, but only faint signal in the endothelium of the muscular PA (original magnification ×200). (*Bottom*) Western blot analysis for eNOS in protein extracts from lung tissue of 2 nonsmokers and 4 smokers, and from a human aortic endothelium cell line (CTL). M, marker; CTL, control. (*From* Barberà JA, Peinado VI, Santos S, et al. Reduced expression of endothelial nitric oxide synthase in pulmonary arteries of smokers. Am J Respir Crit Care Med 2001;164(4):711; with permission.)

oxygen therapy group were nearly double those in the continuous oxygen therapy group (20.6% vs 11.9% after 1 year, and 40.8% vs 22.4% after 2 years). After 6 months of therapy, there was a trend toward lower mPAP and PVR in patients who used oxygen continuously compared with those who used it only at night. The results of the Medical Research Council and Nocturnal Oxygen Therapy Trial studies do not exclude improvements in pulmonary hemodynamics as the mechanism by which LTo_2 prolongs survival. However, to date, proof of this hypothesis is lacking. Nonetheless, oxygen remains a vital part of therapy for PH in patients with COPD.

The use of vasodilator medications to treat PH associated with COPD has been complicated by their effect on oxygenation. These agents may impede gas exchange by inhibiting the primary mechanism by which the lung matches perfusion to ventilation. Earlier studies with systemic vasodilators such as calcium channel blockers or hydralazine have not shown sustained benefit and blunt hypoxic pulmonary vasoconstriction, thereby worsening V/Q matching (for review see Ref.[71]). With the development of more selective pulmonary vasodilators for the treatment of PAH, interest in pharmacologic therapy for PH in chronic lung disease has increased. Although these agents have the same inhibitory effect on hypoxic

pulmonary vasoconstriction, many also have antiproliferative, antiinflammatory, and antifibrotic properties that seem well suited for treating COPD and ILD as well. Early case reports and small single-center studies offered encouraging results to support this idea. However, larger clinical trials have not found consistent beneficial effects. Part of the challenge has been to identify the group of patients with chronic lung disease that is most likely to benefit from medical treatment of their PH. Lowering PAP in patients with moderate PH and severe lung disease may not be of any benefit because the patients will still have significant ventilator impairment. In contrast, patients with severe PH and mild to moderate lung disease may derive greater benefit than those with moderate PH if they represent a unique phenotype characterized by more pulmonary vascular disease than airways disease.

In order to better understand how each therapy affects PH in chronic lung disease, clinical trials in this article have been divided into 3 categories (**Table 1**): (1) chronic lung disease with no PH or mild PH. These studies addressed the effect of PAH-specific medications on COPD or ILD regardless of the presence or absence of PH. (2) Chronic lung disease with moderate PH. These studies assessed PAP and required patients to have PH as part of their entry criteria, but made no effort

Table 1
Studies of PH-specific medications in patient with chronic lung disease and variable degree of PH

	ERA	PDE5I	Prostanoid	NO and sGC+
COPD mild or no PH	Stolz et al,[72] 2008	Lederer et al,[75] 2012 Rao 2011[107]	—	—
COPD moderate PH	Valerio et al,[73] 2009	Alp et al,[76] 2006 Madden et al,[77] 2006 Holverda et al,[78] 2008 Blanco et al,[79,81] 2010, 2013 Rietema et al,[80] 2008	—	Vonbank et al,[84] 2003 Ghofrani et al,[85] 2015
COPD severe PH	Badesch et al,[74] 2012	—	Dernaika et al,[82] 2010	—
ILD mild or no PH	King et al,[86,87] 2008, 2011 Raghu et al,[88,89] 2013, 2013	Zisman et al,[91] 2010 Jackson et al,[92] 2010	—	—
ILD moderate PH	Corte et al,[90] 2014	Han et al,[95] 2013 Ghofrani et al,[93] 2002 Corte et al,[94] 2010	—	Hoeper et al,[99] 2013
ILD severe PH	Badesch et al,[74] 2012	Zimmerman et al,[96] 2014	Saggar et al,[98] 2014	—

Abbreviations: ERA, endothelin receptor antagonist; PDE5I, phosphodiesterase type-5 inhibitor; sGC+, soluble guanylate cyclase stimulator.

to select out patients with severe PH and thus the average mPAP is in a moderate range of approximately 25 to 35 mm Hg. (3) Chronic lung disease with severe PH. These studies examined the effect of PAH-specific therapy on patients with chronic lung disease and severe PH, with mPAP usually greater than 40 mm Hg. Clinical trials have not been conducted with all PAH-specific medications for each group described above and many of the studies that have been done are small and unblinded, but the groupings in **Table 1** help to organize what has been done and gives the reader a view of what studies are needed.

Endothelin receptor antagonist for pulmonary hypertension associated with chronic obstructive pulmonary disease

One of the first randomized controlled trials (RCTs) to examine the effect of PAH-specific medications on chronic lung disease studied the effect of the nonselective endothelin receptor antagonist (ERA) bosentan in 30 patients with moderate to severe COPD.[72] The primary outcome variable was change from baseline in 6-minute walk distance (6MWD). Twenty patients were randomized to bosentan and 10 to placebo. Although two-thirds of the subjects were reported to have PH measured by TTE, the group that received bosentan had a median right ventricle to right atrial systolic pressure gradient that was at the upper limit of normal at 32 mm Hg and FEV_1 was 38% ± 13% predicted. After 12 weeks of treatment, 6MWD remained unchanged in those given placebo (331 ± 116 m at baseline vs 331 ± 123 m at week 12; $P = .100$) and decreased 10 m in patients treated with bosentan (339 ± 81 m at baseline to 329 ± 94 m at week 12; $P = .040$). At the same time, Pao_2 decreased from 65.2 ± 10.5 mm Hg to 60.7 ± 7.5 mm Hg ($P<.05$) and the median alveolar-arterial oxygen gradient increased from 31.4 (28.1–37.1) mm Hg to 40.4 (31.5–44.9) mm Hg in the bosentan group, whereas both of these measures were unchanged in patients given placebo. There was no change in lung function or PAP as measured by PFTs and transthoracic echocardiogram, respectively, but quality of life as assessed by the Short-form-36 Health Survey decreased significantly in the patients assigned to bosentan.

In a similar-sized study, 32 patients with the same degree of COPD as in the study above (mean FEV_1 37% ± 18%) but with moderate PH (mPAP 37 ± 5 mm Hg) were randomized in unblinded fashion to best respiratory care plus placebo or bosentan.[73] After 18 months of treatment, patients who received bosentan had a significant improvement in mPAP from 37 ± 5 mm Hg to 31 ± 6 mm Hg and PVR from 442 ± 192 dyn/s/cm⁵ to 392 ± 180 dyn/s/cm⁵. The 6MWD increased from 256 ± 118 m to 321 ± 122 m. Although the results of this unblinded study suggest that ERAs may be of benefit in the treatment of COPD with moderate to severe PH, limited data from the ARIES-3 study do not suggest that this is true. In that study, 24 patients with more modest COPD (FEV_1 ≥50% predicted) and more severe PH (mPAP ≥45 mm Hg) treated with the selective ERA ambrisentan at a dose of 5 mg daily had a mean decrease in 6MWD of 5 m (95% confidence interval [CI], −34–24) after 24 weeks of treatment.[74]

Phosphodiesterase inhibitors for pulmonary hypertension associated with chronic obstructive pulmonary disease

The use of phosphodiesterase type-5 (PDE5) inhibitors also does not seem to be warranted in patients with COPD who do not have PH. In one small study,[75] 10 patients with COPD were randomized to 4 weeks of sildenafil or placebo followed by a 1-week washout and then 4 weeks of the opposite treatment using a crossover design. Sildenafil had no effect on 6MWD or oxygen consumption at peak exercise, but significantly increased the alveolar-arterial oxygen gradient and the frequency of adverse events and decreased quality of life. Interest in using PDE5 inhibitors in patients with COPD with PH was generated in part by favorable reports from small open-label studies.[76,77] For example, Alp and colleagues[76] studied 6 patients with severe COPD and moderate PH measured by RHC. Twelve weeks after starting treatment with sildenafil (50 mg twice daily), mPAP decreased from 30.2 ± 5.5 mm Hg to 24.6 ± 4.2 mm Hg and the 6MWD increased from 351 ± 49 m to 433 ± 52 m. However, larger studies did not suggest that PDE5 inhibitors are helpful in these patients. In 2 studies that examined the acute effect of sildenafil on pulmonary hemodynamics and oxygenation in patients with COPD with and without PH, sildenafil was found to reduce PAP during exercise but with minimal or no improvement in CO.[78,79] In the first study, Helveroda and colleagues[78] found that sildenafil reduced the exercise-induced increase in mPAP without worsening gas exchange, but there was no increase in stroke volume, CO, or maximal exercise. In the other study, Blanco and colleagues[79] examined the acute effect of sildenafil on pulmonary hemodynamics and gas exchange in 20 patients with COPD, 17 of whom had mPAP greater than 17 mm Hg at rest. Sildenafil significantly reduced mPAP and oxygenation at rest. The decrease in oxygenation was caused by an increase in perfusion to areas of low V/Q consistent with the concept that sildenafil worsened oxygenation by blunting hypoxic pulmonary vasoconstriction in areas of decreased ventilation (**Fig. 8**). During moderate exercise, sildenafil reduced mPAP without worsening oxygenation and resulted in a slight increase in CO; however, there was no improvement in oxygen delivery. These acute studies suggest that sildenafil has favorable hemodynamic effects and is well tolerated but it is unclear whether improvement in hemodynamics can result in improved exercise capacity.

In a study designed to determine whether sildenafil could increase stroke volume during exercise and improve functional capacity, Rietema and colleagues[80] treated 15 patients with Global Initiative for Chronic Obstructive Lung Disease (GOLD) stage II to IV COPD with sildenafil for 12 weeks. PH was assessed by RHC and stroke volume was measured by MRI at rest and during submaximal exercise. Nine patients were found to have PH. Compared with healthy controls, stroke volume in patients with COPD was significantly lower at rest (62 ± 12 mL vs 81 ± 22 mL) and during exercise (70 ± 15 mL vs 101 ± 28 mL). After 12 weeks of treatment with sildenafil (50 mg 3 times daily), there was no change from baseline in stroke volume at rest or during exercise and no significant improvement in 6MWD regardless of the presence or absence of PH.

In addition, in a larger RCT of 63 patients with COPD and PH diagnosed by TTE, sildenafil was found to have no effect on exercise capacity during 3 months of cardiopulmonary exercise training.[81] In this important study, patients were randomized in double-blind fashion to sildenafil 20 mg 3 times a day or placebo before 3 months of supervised cardiopulmonary training. At the end of the study, cycle endurance time increased

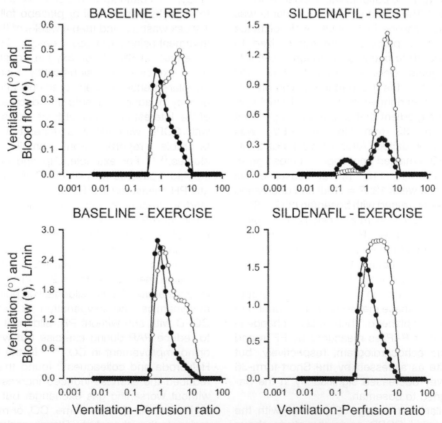

Fig. 8. Ventilation-perfusion (VA/Q) distributions at rest and during exercise, before and after sildenafil in a patient with COPD. The amount of ventilation (*open circles*) and blood flow (*solid circles*) in units with a different VA/Q ratio in each study condition is shown. At rest there is a shift in blood flow to units with low VA/Q ratio after administration of sildenafil. No change in VA/Q distributions was observed after sildenafil during exercise (*bottom*). (*From* Blanco I, Gimeno E, Munoz PA, et al. Hemodynamic and gas exchange effects of sildenafil in patients with chronic obstructive pulmonary disease and pulmonary hypertension. Am J Respir Crit Care Med 2010;181:273; with permission.)

149 seconds in patients who received sildenafil and 169 seconds in those given placebo, and the 6MWD increased 23 and 21 meters (m), respectively. There were slight gains in the quality-of-life scores, which did not differ between study groups.

Prostacyclin analogues for treatment of pulmonary hypertension associated with chronic obstructive pulmonary disease

Few studies have examined the effect of prostacyclin derivatives for treating PH associated with COPD. One potential advantage is that they are available as inhalational agents and by this route could avoid much of the inhibitor effect that orally or intravenously administered medications have on hypoxic pulmonary vasoconstriction. In a small study of 10 patients with COPD and severe PH (mPAP >40 mm Hg) iloprost improved 6MWD from 269 ± 112 m at baseline to 330 ± 136 m measured 3 minutes after the second dose of iloprost.[82] Iloprost had no effect on oxygenation, systemic blood pressure, spirometry, or DLco. The 6MWD returned to baseline 2 hours after the last treatment. However, no studies have evaluated the long-term effect of inhaled prostacyclins on PH in COPD.

Soluble guanylate cyclase stimulators for pulmonary hypertension associated with chronic obstructive pulmonary disease

Inhaled NO (iNO) and the newly developed soluble guanylate cyclase (sGC) stimulators such as riociguat cause pulmonary vasodilation by increasing cyclic GMP (cGMP) levels. In addition, sGC stimulators have been shown to prevent cigarette smoke–induced PH and emphysema in animal models of lung disease.[83] Few data are available regarding the use of these agents to treat PH associated with COPD. However, in one well-designed RCT, 48 patients with moderate PH caused by COPD were randomly assigned to receive supplemental oxygen alone or in combination with pulsed inhalation of NO for 3 months.[84] In patients who were given iNO, there was a significant decrease in mPAP from 27.6 ± 4.4 mm Hg to 20.6 ± 4.9 mm Hg ($P<.001$) and PVRi from 570 ± 208 dyn/s/cm^5/m^2 to 351 ± 160 dyn/s/cm^5/m^2 ($P<.001$), and an increase in CO from 5.6 ± 1.3 L/min to 6.1 ± 1.0 L/min ($P = .025$). Systemic hemodynamics, oxygenation, and PFTs did not change significantly. Subjective improvement in physical performance as assessed by questionnaire increased by 38.5% in patients given iNO compared with 12.5% in patients treated with oxygen alone ($P = .047$). Although these data were encouraging, the lack of development of a practical iNO delivery device has prevented this

therapy from becoming available. A more reasonable approach to stimulating cGMP production in patients with COPD may be the use of sGC stimulators. In a recently reported pilot study,[85] patients with COPD and moderate PH were given riociguat at a dose of 1.0 mg (n = 10) or 2.5 mg (n = 12) during RHC. A decrease in mPAP of 11.4% and 14.8% and in PVR of 15.3% and 33.0% were reported for the 1.0-mg and 2.5-mg doses, respectively. No adverse effects on oxygenation were seen. A clinical trial of riociguat in PH associated with COPD is currently being considered.

At present the available data do not support the use of PAH-specific medications for the treatment of PH associated with COPD. Data on the use of ERAs in COPD are limited and conflicting. Unconfirmed results of small open-label studies suggest that PDE5 inhibitors, inhaled prostacyclin, or sGC stimulators may have acute beneficial effects in select patients, but extended benefits have not been shown in randomized prospective studies.

Treatment of pulmonary hypertension Associated with interstitial lung disease

Endothelin receptor antagonists for pulmonary hypertension in interstitial lung disease

There has been considerable interest in both the ERAs and PDE5 inhibitor (PDE5I) in the treatment of ILD without PH because of the known antifibrotic and antiinflammatory properties of these agents. All 3 presently available ERAs have been studied in ILD. The first study examined the effect of the nonselective ERA bosentan on 158 patients with IPF randomly assigned to receive bosentan or placebo.[86] No difference was seen in the primary end point of change in 6MWD up to month 12. A trend in favor of bosentan was seen in a secondary end point of time to death or disease progression, which was more pronounced in a subgroup of patients who had been diagnosed by surgical lung biopsy. However, a larger follow-up study[87] of 616 patients randomized 2:1 to bosentan or placebo found no significant effect of bosentan on IPF worsening, exacerbation of IPF, or death.

Another study examined the effect of ambrisentan, which has greater selectivity for the endothelin A receptor than bosentan, on the time to disease progression, defined as death, respiratory hospitalization, or decrease in lung function, in 492 patients with IPF, 10% of whom had PH.[88] The study was stopped after only 75% of intended enrollment because an interim analysis indicated a low likelihood of efficacy. Ambrisentan-treated patients were more likely to meet the criteria for disease progression (27.4% vs 17.2%; $P<.010$; hazard ratio, 1.74 [95% CI, 1.14–2.66]) and had more hospitalizations (13.4% vs 5.5%; P<.007) after a mean duration of exposure to the study drug of 34.7 weeks. There were also trends toward greater decline in lung function (16.7% vs 11.7%; P<.109) and death (7.9% vs 3.7%; P<.100) in the ambrisentan-treated patients.

In the same year, the effect of macitentan, a newly developed nonselective ERA with a very high receptor occupancy half-life, was reported in 178 subjects with IPF who were randomized (2:1) to macitentan (n = 119) or placebo (n = 59).[89] The median change from baseline up to month 12 in forced vital capacity was −0.20 L in both the macitentan and the placebo arms. There were no differences between treatment groups in FEV_1, DLco, or time to disease worsening or death.

These studies showed the lack of efficacy of ERAs in patients with IPF in the absence of significant PH. However, few studies have examined the effect of ERAs in patients with ILD and PH. In one of the few studies that have, 60 patients with idiopathic interstitial pneumonia and PH confirmed by RHC were randomized 2:1 to treatment with bosentan (n = 40) or placebo (n = 20) for 16 weeks[90]. The mPAP was 36.0 ± 8.9 mm Hg, mean PVRi was 13.0 ± 6.7 Wood units/m^2, and mean cardiac index was 2.21 ± 0.5 L/min/m^2 indicating severe PH. The primary study end point, defined as a decrease from baseline in PVRi of greater than or equal to 20%, did not differ between treatment groups, occurring in 28.0% of patients given bosentan and 28.6% of patient assigned to placebo (**Fig. 9**). The 6MWD decreased 25.9 ± 56.7 m and 53.1 ± 66.9 m in the bosentan and placebo groups respectively. No change in symptoms, rates of serious adverse events, or deaths were seen between the two groups.

A similar lack of efficacy was reported in the ARIES-3 study, which examined the efficacy and safety of ambrisentan in patients with PH of various causes using an open-label design.[74] There were 21 patients with ILD who were treated with ambrisentan for 24 weeks. The mean mPAP and PVR in this group were 41 ± 7 mm Hg and 6.8 ± 2.6 mm Hg/L/min, respectively. The mean change from baseline in 6MWD at week 24 decreased 23 m (95% CI, −60–14 m). This finding is similar to the 26 m decrease in 6MWD that was seen in the bosentan study and suggests that ERAs are not helpful at improving functional capacity in patients with PH associated with ILD.

Phosphodiesterase inhibitors for pulmonary hypertension associated with interstitial lung disease

In 2010, Zisman and colleagues[91] reported the results of a randomized placebo-controlled study of 180 patients with IPF treated with sildenafil. PH was not included in the entry criteria for this study, but echocardiographic measurements of PAP were available for slightly more than a third of the patients studied. In these patients, the mean RVSP was 42.5 mm Hg, suggesting a mild to moderate degree of PH. The primary outcome variable was the number of patients who achieved a 20% improvement in 6MWD by week 12. There was no difference seen between treatment groups, with 10% of patients in the sildenafil group and 7% in the placebo group achieving an improvement of 20% or more (P = .39). There were small but significant improvements in arterial oxygenation, DLco, degree of dyspnea, and quality of life in the sildenafil group. A smaller study published in the same year[92] also reported no difference in 6MWD between 29 patients with IPF randomized to sildenafil (n = 15) or placebo (n = 14). After 6 months of

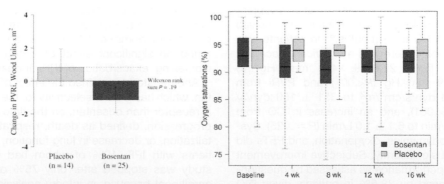

Fig. 9. (*Left*) Absolute change in PVRi after 16 weeks in patients treated with bosentan or placebo. (*Right*) Change in arterial oxygen saturations, measured every 4 weeks, from baseline to week 16 in the same study cohort. (*From* Corte TJ, Keir GJ, Dimopoulos K, et al; BPHIT Study Group. Bosentan in pulmonary hypertension associated with fibrotic idiopathic interstitial pneumonia. Am J Respir Crit Care Med 2014;190(2):213; with permission.)

treatment the mean 6MWD was 324 ± 41 m in the sildenafil group versus 355 ± 82 m in patients given placebo (P = .256). There were also no differences in changes in mean Borg score (sildenafil 4.1 ± 2.3 vs placebo 3.4 ± 1.6; P = .492). Sildenafil had no effect on RVSP, which was at the upper limit of normal, or on oxygenation or decrease in oxygenation with exercise.

Few studies have examined the effect of PDE5I on patients with ILD and moderate PH. In 2002, Ghofranhi and colleagues[93] reported an acute decrease of greater than 20% in PVR in response to iNO, sildenafil, or epoprostenol in 16 patients hospitalized with pulmonary fibrosis and PH. The ratio of pulmonary to systemic vascular resistance decreased only in patients given iNO or sildenafil and only iNO and sildenafil improved V/Q ratio and oxygenation, suggesting that, in this population, a PDE5I may be beneficial. Corte and colleagues[94] presented a retrospective review on 15 patients with various forms of ILD and PH who were treated with sildenafil. The mPAP in 11 patients who underwent RHC was 41.3 + 11 mm Hg at baseline. However, no change in RVSP as assessed by TTE in 11 of the patients was seen and only 6 of the 15 patients examined completed the follow-up 6MWD test at the end of the 6-month treatment. Four of these 6 patients had an improvement in 6MWD.

In a substudy from the IPFnet trial described earlier[91] in which 180 patients with IPF were randomized to sildenafil or placebo, Han and colleagues[95] examined the effect of sildenafil on right ventricular (RV) function in those patients who had PH and found 119 patients who had echocardiograms available for review. Of these patients, echocardiographic evidence of RVH and RV systolic dysfunction was seen in 12.8% and 18.6%, respectively. The RVSP could be estimated in 60% of the subjects and mean RVSP was 42.5 mm Hg. In patients with no evidence of RVH or RV dysfunction, there was no change in 6MWD after 12 weeks in those randomized to sildenafil or placebo. In patients with evidence of RVH or RV dysfunction, the 6MWD decreased in those given placebo, but not in those randomized to receive sildenafil. For the group with RV dysfunction, the mean difference in 6MWD at 12 weeks was 99 m. These findings suggest that although sildenafil does not improve 6MWD in patients with ILD with PH, it may prevent 6MWD from decreasing if there is evidence of RV dysfunction on echocardiogram.

Recently, Zimmerman and colleagues[96] reported an improvement in mPAP and PVR in 10 patients with ILD and severe PH treated with either sildenafil or tadalafil for a mean duration of

6.9 ± 5.8 months. In this uncontrolled, open-label study, there was a decrease in PVR from 519 ± 131 dyn/s/cm^5 to 403 ± 190 dyn/s/cm^5 (P = .04) and a trend toward a decrease in mPAP from 42.9 ± 5.4 mm Hg at baseline to 36.1 ± 7.6 mm Hg (P = .07), but there was no change in 6MWD (290 ± 82.3 m vs 293.3 ± 78.4 m; P = .87) or brain natriuretic peptide level (247 ± 212 ng/mL vs 296 ± 353 ng/mL).

Prostacyclin derivatives for pulmonary hypertension associated with interstitial lung disease

There are few trials of prostacyclin derivatives in the treatment of PH associated with ILD. A case report of a patient with severe usual interstitial pneumonitis who improved with intravenous treprostinil while awaiting lung transplant generated some interest in whether this therapy could provide benefit to patients with severe PH and ILD.[97] In 2014, the same group reported their experience with 15 patients with pulmonary fibrosis and advanced PH defined as mPAP greater than or equal to 35 mm Hg who were treated with 12 weeks of parenteral treprostinil while awaiting lung transplant.[98] At the end of the study period, right atrial pressure decreased from 9.5 ± 3.4 mm Hg to 6.0 ± 3.7 mm Hg, mPAP decreased from 47 ± 8 mm Hg to 38.9 ± 13.4 mm Hg, cardiac index increased from 2.3 ± 0.5 L/min/m^2 to 2.7 ± 0.6 L/min/m^2, and PVR decreased from 698 ± 278 dyn/cm/s^5 to 496 ± 229 dyn/cm/s^5. Right ventricle function improved, as shown by a decrease in RV end-diastolic area from 36.4 ± 5.2 cm^2 to 30.9 ± 8.2 cm^2 and an increase in the tricuspid annular planar systolic excursion from 1.6 ± 0.5 cm to 1.9 ± 0.2 cm. No significant change in systemic oxygenation or mean systemic arterial pressure was seen and there were significant improvements in 6MWD (171 ± 93 m vs 230 ± 114 m); 36-Item Short-form Health Survey Mental Component Summary aggregate (38 ± 11 vs 44.2 ± 10.7); University of California, San Diego Shortness of Breath Questionnaire (87 ± 17.1 vs 73.1 ± 21); and brain natriuretic peptide level (558 ± 859 pg/mL vs 228 ± 340 pg/mL). These impressive findings suggest that intravenous prostacyclin therapy may improve severe PH in some patients with advanced lung disease; however, prospective, controlled studies will be needed to confirm these findings.

Soluble guanylate cyclase stimulators for pulmonary hypertension and interstitial lung disease

No studies have reported the effect of iNO on PH in ILD. One open-label, uncontrolled pilot trial has been completed using the sGC stimulator riociguat.[99] Twenty-two patients with PH caused by ILD were given riociguat (1.0–2.5 mg 3 times daily) for 12 weeks, followed by an extension study. After 12 weeks of therapy, mean CO increased from 4.4 ± 1.5 L/min to 5.5 ± 1.8 L/min, PVR decreased from 648 ± 207 dyn/s/cm^5 to 528 ± 181 dyn/s/cm^5, and mPAP was unchanged from baseline. The 6MWD increased from 325 ± 96 m to 351 ± 111 m. However, there were 8 adverse effects that were thought to be drug related and arterial oxygen saturation decreased slightly. A randomized, double-blind, placebo-controlled, phase II study of the safety and efficacy of riociguat in patients with PH associated with idiopathic interstitial pneumonias (clinicaltrials.gov) was recently terminated after observing that patients given riociguat were at a possibly increased risk of serious adverse events compared to placebo.

At present the available data do not support the use of ERA for the treatment of PH associated with ILD. Unconfirmed results of small open-label studies suggest that PDE5 inhibitors, sGC stimulators, or intravenous prostacyclins may have beneficial effects in select patients, but the treatment effect seems to be small and adverse events have been reported. Further studies are needed to confirm these findings.

Treatment of Pulmonary Hypertension Associated with Sleep Disordered Breathing

Unlike COPD and ILD, SDB is usually a treatable condition. Several studies have shown that noninvasive ventilation using continuous positive airway pressure (CPAP) or bilevel positive airway pressure can effectively prevent the apneas and hypopneas that occur during sleep and the decrease in oxygen saturation that accompanies it. The regular use of noninvasive positive pressure ventilation (NIPPV) has also been shown to reverse daytime hypoxia and hypercapnia; decrease circulating levels of ET-1, IL-6, and C-reactive protein[100]; improve vascular endothelial function; and decrease platelet activation and aggregation.[101] CPAP has therefore been shown to be effective at decreasing PAP in patients with SDB and PH. In a study of 20 patients with OSA in which other causes of PH, such as cardiac disease, systemic hypertension, and COPD, had been excluded, 4 months of CPAP reduced mPAP from 16.8 + 1.2 mm Hg to 13.9 + 0.6 mm Hg (P<.05).[102] More importantly, in the 5 patients who had PH defined as mPAP greater than 20 mm Hg before starting CPAP, mPAP returned to within the normal range by the end of the study. In another study, 23 patients with OSA, 10 of whom had PH defined as sPAP greater than 30 mm Hg by TTE, were randomized

to CPAP or sham CPAP for 3 months and then switched to the other therapy in a crossover design for an additional 3 months.[103] There was a significant reduction in PAP during the CPAP arm, with the greatest reduction in the patients with PH (Fig. 10). Extended treatment with CPAP has been shown not only to decrease PAP but to increase circulating levels of NO metabolites and decrease the acute pulmonary vasoconstrictive response to hypoxia.[104]

The efficacy of NIPPV in treating OSA, as well as its beneficial effect on reducing PAP, usually precludes the use of PAH-specific medications to treat PH associated with SDB. Some patients with severe OSA or OHS require tracheostomy with or without nocturnal ventilation to control their sleep apnea. Although it may seem less invasive or more convenient to treat PH associated with uncontrolled SDB with PAH-specific medications rather than proceeding to tracheostomy, adequate control of OSA/OHS has important consequences

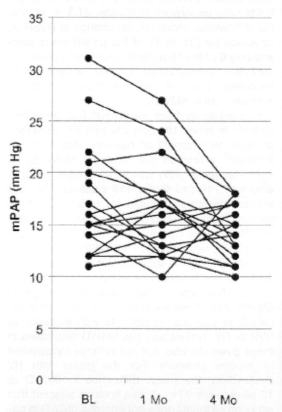

Fig. 10. Effect of 4 months of CPAP on mPAP in 20 patients with obstructive sleep apnea. Note the greatest reduction in mPAP is seen in those who had PH at the start of the study. BL, baseline. (*From* Sajkov D, Wang T, Saunders NA, et al. Continuous positive airway pressure treatment improves pulmonary hemodynamics in patients with obstructive sleep apnea. Am J Respir Crit Care Med 2002;165(2):154; with permission.)

on long-term health because it significantly reduces the risk of systemic hypertension, congestive heart failure, and cerebrovascular accident. Therefore, unless a patient is in danger of overt right heart failure, every attempt should be made to correct the underlying SDB before considering PAH-specific medications to treat PH associated with OSA or OHS. For most patients, PH should be assessed before treatment of their SDB and then again after 3 to 4 months of effective NIPPV designed from the results of CPAP titration and confirmed by home monitoring. Adequate control of a patient's SDB, indicated by the lack of nocturnal oxygen desaturation and daytime hypoxia or hypercapnia, should be achieved before considering the use of PAH-specific medications. For patients who have persistent PH despite adequate control of their SDB, pulmonary vasodilator therapy may be indicated following standard treatment guidelines for WHO group 1 PAH.[105,106]

SUMMARY

PH is common in chronic lung diseases such as COPD, ILD, and OSA. When present, it is usually moderate and correlates with the severity of the underlying lung disease. A small minority of patients have PH that is severe, with mPAP that approaches values seen in patients with PAH. These patients often have moderate or even mild reduction in lung function, but severe reduction in DLco. These patients may represent a different phenotype characterized by greater pulmonary vascular disease. The presence of PH is associated with increased morbidity and mortality. Treatment of PH in chronic lung disease should be focused first on treatment of the underlying lung disease. Supplemental oxygen should be used to keep arterial oxygen saturation above a level that can increase pulmonary vascular tone. Bronchodilators and nocturnal ventilation should be used to control hypercapnia and diuretics should be used to control right heart failure. If PH persists despite optimal management of the underlying lung disease it may be reasonable to consider pulmonary vasodilatory therapy in patients with severe PH associated with mild to moderate disease, usually in consultation with a center that is experienced in the management of PAH. Medications that are currently approved for the treatment of PAH have not been well studied in PH associated with chronic lung disease but the limited data available do not suggest sustained benefit. Considering the large number of patients who have PH associated with chronic lung disease, it is hoped that future studies will identify new targets for treatment of PH in chronic lung disease and continue to attempt to define which patients are most likely to benefit.

REFERENCES

1. Strange G, Playford D, Stewart S, et al. Pulmonary hypertension: prevalence and mortality in the Armadale echocardiography cohort. Heart 2012; 98(24):1805–11.
2. Badesch DB, Champion HC, Sanchez MA, et al. Diagnosis and assessment of pulmonary arterial hypertension. J Am Coll Cardiol 2009;54(Suppl 1):S55–66.
3. Raeside DA, Brown A, Patel KR, et al. Ambulatory pulmonary artery pressure monitoring during sleep and exercise in normal individuals and patients with COPD. Thorax 2002;57(12):1050–3.
4. Lam CS, Borlaug BA, Kane GC, et al. Age-associated increases in pulmonary artery systolic pressure in the general population. Circulation 2009; 119(20):2663–70.
5. D'Alonzo GE, Barst RJ, Ayres SM, et al. Survival in patients with primary pulmonary hypertension. Results from a national prospective registry. Ann Intern Med 1991;115(5):343–9.
6. Humbert M, Sitbon O, Chaouat A, et al. Survival in patients with idiopathic, familial, and anorexigen-associated pulmonary arterial hypertension in the modern management era. Circulation 2010; 122(2):156–63.
7. Badesch DB, Raskob GE, Elliott CG, et al. Pulmonary arterial hypertension: baseline characteristics from the REVEAL Registry. Chest 2010; 137(2):376–87.
8. Chatila WM, Thomashow BM, Minai OA, et al. Comorbidities in chronic obstructive pulmonary disease. Proc Am Thorac Soc 2008;5(4):549–55.
9. Falk JA, Kadiev S, Criner GJ, et al. Cardiac disease in chronic obstructive pulmonary disease. Proc Am Thorac Soc 2008;5(4):543–8.
10. Chaouat A, Naeije R, Weitzenblum E. Pulmonary hypertension in COPD. Eur Respir J 2008;32(5): 1371–85.
11. Arcasoy SM, Christie JD, Ferrari VA, et al. Echocardiographic assessment of pulmonary hypertension in patients with advanced lung disease. Am J Respir Crit Care Med 2003;167(5):735–40.
12. Vizza CD, Lynch JP, Ochoa LL, et al. Right and left ventricular dysfunction in patients with severe pulmonary disease. Chest 1998;113(3):576–83.
13. Thabut G, Dauriat G, Stern JB, et al. Pulmonary hemodynamics in advanced COPD candidates for lung volume reduction surgery or lung transplantation. Chest 2005;127(5):1531–6.
14. Scharf SM, Iqbal M, Keller C, et al, National Emphysema Treatment Trial (NETT) Group. Hemodynamic characterization of patients with severe

emphysema. Am J Respir Crit Care Med 2002; 166(3):314–22.

15. Cuttica MJ, Kalhan R, Shlobin OA, et al. Categorization and impact of pulmonary hypertension in patients with advanced COPD. Respir Med 2010; 104(12):1877–82.

16. Weitzenblum E, Hirth C, Ducolone A, et al. Prognostic value of pulmonary artery pressure in chronic obstructive pulmonary disease. Thorax 1981;36(10):752–8.

17. Doi M, Nakano K, Hiramoto T, et al. Significance of pulmonary artery pressure in emphysema patients with mild-to moderate hypoxemia. Respir Med 2003;97(8):915–20.

18. Burrows B, Kettel LJ, Niden AH, et al. Patterns of cardiovascular dysfunction in chronic obstructive lung disease. N Engl J Med 1972;286(17):912–8.

19. Higham MA, Dawson D, Joshi J, et al. Utility of echocardiography in assessment of pulmonary hypertension secondary to COPD. Eur Respir J 2001; 17(3):350–5.

20. Fayngersh V, Drakopanagiotakis F, Dennis McCool F, et al. Pulmonary hypertension in a stable community-based COPD population. Lung 2011; 189(5):377–82.

21. Oswald-Mammosser M, Apprill M, Bachez P, et al. Pulmonary hemodynamics in chronic obstructive pulmonary disease of the emphysematous type. Respiration 1991;58(5–6):304–10.

22. Christensen CC, Ryg MS, Edvardsen A, et al. Relationship between exercise desaturation and pulmonary haemodynamics in COPD patients. Eur Respir J 2004;24(4):580–6.

23. Fujimoto K, Matsuzawa Y, Yamaguchi S, et al. Benefits of oxygen on exercise performance and pulmonary hemodynamics in patients with COPD with mild hypoxemia. Chest 2002;122(2):457–63.

24. Kessler R, Faller M, Weitzenblum E, et al. "Natural history" of pulmonary hypertension in a series of 131 patients with chronic obstructive lung disease. Am J Respir Crit Care Med 2001;164(2):219–24.

25. Lettieri CJ, Nathan SD, Barnett SD, et al. Prevalence and outcomes of pulmonary arterial hypertension in advanced idiopathic pulmonary fibrosis. Chest 2006;129(3):746–52.

26. Shorr AF, Wainright JL, Cors CS, et al. Pulmonary hypertension in patients with pulmonary fibrosis awaiting lung transplant. Eur Respir J 2007;30(4): 715–21.

27. Nathan SD, Shlobin OA, Ahmad S, et al. Pulmonary hypertension and pulmonary function testing in idiopathic pulmonary fibrosis. Chest 2007;131(3): 657–63.

28. Lederer DJ, Arcasoy SM, Wilt JS, et al. Six-minute-walk distance predicts waiting list survival in idiopathic pulmonary fibrosis. Am J Respir Crit Care Med 2006;174(6):659–64.

29. Patel NM, Lederer DJ, Borczuk AC, et al. Pulmonary hypertension in idiopathic pulmonary fibrosis. Chest 2007;132(3):998–1006.

30. Taraseviciute A, Voelkel NF. Severe pulmonary hypertension in postmenopausal obese women. Eur J Med Res 2006;11(5):198–202.

31. Zamanian RT, Hansmann G, Snook S, et al. Insulin resistance in pulmonary arterial hypertension. Eur Respir J 2009;33(2):318–24.

32. Ismail K, Roberts K, Manning P, et al. OSA and pulmonary hypertension: time for a new look. Chest 2015;147(3):847–61.

33. Minai OA, Ricaurte B, Kaw R, et al. Frequency and impact of pulmonary hypertension in patients with obstructive sleep apnea syndrome. Am J Cardiol 2009;104(9):1300–6.

34. Chaouat A, Weitzenblum E, Krieger J, et al. Pulmonary hemodynamics in the obstructive sleep apnea syndrome. Results in 220 consecutive patients. Chest 1996;109(2):380–6.

35. Kessler R, Chaouat A, Schinkewitch P, et al. The obesity hypoventilation syndrome revisited: a prospective study of 34 consecutive cases. Chest 2001;120(2):369–76.

36. Sugerman HJ, Baron PL, Fairman RP, et al. Hemodynamic dysfunction in obesity hypoventilation syndrome and the effects of treatment with surgically induced weight loss. Ann Surg 1988;207(5): 604–13.

37. Chaouat A, Bugnet AS, Kadaoui N, et al. Severe pulmonary hypertension and chronic obstructive pulmonary disease. Am J Respir Crit Care Med 2005;172(2):189–94.

38. Hurdman J, Condliffe R, Elliot CA, et al. Pulmonary hypertension in COPD: results from the ASPIRE registry. Eur Respir J 2013;41:1292–301.

39. Oswald-Mammosser M, Weitzenblum E, Quoix E, et al. Prognostic factors in COPD patients receiving long-term oxygen therapy. Importance of pulmonary artery pressure. Chest 1995; 107(5):1193–8.

40. Naeije R. Pulmonary hypertension and right heart failure in COPD. Monaldi Arch Chest Dis 2003; 59(3):250–3.

41. Stone AC, Machan JT, Mazer J, et al. Echocardiographic evidence of pulmonary hypertension is associated with increased 1-year mortality in patients admitted with chronic obstructive pulmonary disease. Lung 2011;189(3):207–12.

42. Kessler R, Faller M, Fourgaut G, et al. Predictive factors of hospitalization for acute exacerbation in a series of 64 patients with chronic obstructive pulmonary disease. Am J Respir Crit Care Med 1999; 159(1):158–64.

43. Nadrous HF, Pellikka PA, Krowka MJ, et al. Pulmonary hypertension in patients with idiopathic pulmonary fibrosis. Chest 2005;128(4):2393–9.

44. Hamada K, Nagai S, Tanaka S, et al. Significance of pulmonary arterial pressure and diffusion capacity of the lung as prognosticator in patients with idiopathic pulmonary fibrosis. Chest 2007;131(3): 650–6.

45. Leuchte HH, Neurohr C, Baumgartner R, et al. Brain natriuretic peptide and exercise capacity in lung fibrosis and pulmonary hypertension. Am J Respir Crit Care Med 2004;170(4):360–5.

46. Verma G, Marras T, Chowdhury N, et al. Health-related quality of life and 6 min walk distance in patients with idiopathic pulmonary fibrosis. Can Respir J 2011;18(5):283–7.

47. Harvey RM, Enson Y, Betti R, et al. Further observations on the effect of hydrogen ion on the pulmonary circulation. Circulation 1967;35(6):1019–27.

48. Rudolph AM, Yuan S. Response of the pulmonary vasculature to hypoxia and H+ ion concentration changes. J Clin Invest 1966;45(3):399–411.

49. Fletcher EC, Luckett RA, Miller T, et al. Exercise hemodynamics and gas exchange in patients with chronic obstruction pulmonary disease, sleep desaturation, and a daytime PaO_2 above 60 mm Hg. Am Rev Respir Dis 1989;140(5):1237–45.

50. Grover RF. Chronic hypoxic pulmonary hypertension. In: Fishman AP, editor. The pulmonary circulation: normal and abnormal. Philadelphia: University of Pennsylvania Press; 1990. p. 283–99.

51. Ashutosh K, Mead G, Dunsky M. Early effects of oxygen administration and prognosis in chronic obstructive pulmonary disease and cor pulmonale. Am Rev Respir Dis 1983;127:399–404.

52. Weitzenblum E, Schrijen F, Hohan-Kumar T, et al. Variability of the pulmonary vascular response to acute hypoxia in chronic bronchitis. Chest 1988; 94:772–8.

53. Eddahibi S, Chaouat A, Morrell N, et al. Polymorphism of the serotonin transporter gene and pulmonary hypertension in chronic obstructive pulmonary diseases. Circulation 2003;108: 1839–44.

54. Howell JB, Permutt S, Proctor DF, et al. Effect of inflation of the lung on different parts of pulmonary vascular bed. J Appl Physiol 1961;16:71–6.

55. Colombat M, Mal H, Groussard O, et al. Pulmonary vascular lesions in end-stage idiopathic pulmonary fibrosis: histopathologic study on lung explant specimens and correlations with pulmonary hemodynamics. Hum Pathol 2007;38(1):60–5.

56. Giaid A, Yanagisawa M, Langleben D, et al. Expression of endothelin-1 in the lungs of patients with pulmonary hypertension. N Engl J Med 1993; 328(24):1732–9.

57. Rubens C, Ewert R, Halank M, et al. Big endothelin-1 and endothelin-1 plasma levels are correlated with the severity of primary pulmonary hypertension. Chest 2001;120(5):1562–9.

58. Yamakami T, Taguchi O, Gabazza EC, et al. Arterial endothelin-1 level in pulmonary emphysema and interstitial lung disease. Relation with pulmonary hypertension during exercise. Eur Respir J 1997; 10(9):2055–60.

59. Saleh D, Furukawa K, Tsao MS, et al. Elevated expression of endothelin-1 and endothelin-converting enzyme-1 in idiopathic pulmonary fibrosis: possible involvement of proinflammatory cytokines. Am J Respir Cell Mol Biol 1997;16(2): 187–93.

60. Hocher B, Schwarz A, Fagan KA, et al. Pulmonary fibrosis and chronic lung inflammation in ET-1 transgenic mice. Am J Respir Cell Mol Biol 2000; 23(1):19–26.

61. Steiner MK, Syrkina OL, Kolliputi N, et al. Interleukin-6 overexpression induces pulmonary hypertension. Circ Res 2009;104(2):236–44.

62. Lesur OJ, Mancini NM, Humbert JC, et al. Interleukin-6, interferon-gamma, and phospholipid levels in the alveolar lining fluid of human lungs. Profiles in coal worker's pneumoconiosis and idiopathic pulmonary fibrosis. Chest. 1994;106(2): 407–13.

63. Klinger JR, Abman SH, Gladwin MT. Nitric oxide deficiency and endothelial dysfunction in pulmonary arterial hypertension. Am J Respir Crit Care Med 2013;188(6):639–46.

64. Barberà JA, Peinado VI, Santos S, et al. Reduced expression of endothelial nitric oxide synthase in pulmonary arteries of smokers. Am J Respir Crit Care Med 2001;164(4):709–13.

65. Joppa P, Petrasova D, Stancak B, et al. Systemic inflammation in patients with COPD and pulmonary hypertension. Chest 2006;130(2):326–33.

66. Broekelmann TJ, Limper AH, Colby TV, et al. Transforming growth factor beta 1 is present at sites of extracellular matrix gene expression in human pulmonary fibrosis. Proc Natl Acad Sci U S A 1991; 88(15):6642–6.

67. Morrell NW, Yang X, Upton PD, et al. Altered growth responses of pulmonary artery smooth muscle cells from patients with primary pulmonary hypertension to transforming growth factor-beta(1) and bone morphogenetic proteins. Circulation 2001; 104(7):790–5.

68. Koyama S, Sato E, Haniuda M, et al. Decreased level of vascular endothelial growth factor in bronchoalveolar lavage fluid of normal smokers and patients with pulmonary fibrosis. Am J Respir Crit Care Med 2002;166(3):382–5.

69. Medical Research Council Working Party. Long term domiciliary oxygen therapy in chronic hypoxic cor pulmonale complicating chronic bronchitis and emphysema. Lancet 1981;1:681–6.

70. Nocturnal Oxygen Therapy Trial Group. Continuous or nocturnal oxygen therapy in hypoxemic chronic

obstructive lung disease. Ann Intern Med 1980;93: 391–8.

71. Klinger JR, Hill NS. Right ventricular dysfunction in chronic obstructive pulmonary disease. Evaluation and management. Chest 1991;99(3):715–23.

72. Stolz D, Rasch H, Linka A, et al. A randomised, controlled trial of bosentan in severe COPD. Eur Respir J 2008;32(3):619–28.

73. Valerio G, Bracciale P, Grazia D'Agostino A. Effect of bosentan upon pulmonary hypertension in chronic obstructive pulmonary disease. Ther Adv Respir Dis 2009;3(1):15–21.

74. Badesch DB, Feldman J, Keogh A, et al. ARIES-3: ambrisentan therapy in a diverse population of patients with pulmonary hypertension. Cardiovasc Ther 2012;30(2):93–9.

75. Lederer DJ, Bartels MN, Schluger NW, et al. Sildenafil for chronic obstructive pulmonary disease: a randomized crossover trial. COPD 2012;9(3): 268–75.

76. Alp S, Skrygan M, Schmidt WE, et al. Sildenafil improves hemodynamic parameters in COPD–an investigation of six patients. Pulm Pharmacol Ther 2006;19(6):386–90.

77. Madden BP, Allenby M, Loke TK, et al. A potential role for sildenafil in the management of pulmonary hypertension in patients with parenchymal lung disease. Vascul Pharmacol 2006;44(5):372–6.

78. Holverda S, Rietema H, Bogaard HJ, et al. Acute effects of sildenafil on exercise pulmonary hemodynamics and capacity in patients with COPD. Pulm Pharmacol Ther 2008;21:558–64.

79. Blanco I, Gimeno E, Munoz PA, et al. Hemodynamic and gas exchange effects of sildenafil in patients with chronic obstructive pulmonary disease and pulmonary hypertension. Am J Respir Crit Care Med 2010;181:270–8.

80. Rietema H, Holverda S, Bogaard HJ, et al. Sildenafil treatment in COPD does not affect stroke volume or exercise capacity. Eur Respir J 2008;31: 759–64.

81. Blanco I, Santos S, Gea J, et al. Sildenafil to improve respiratory rehabilitation outcomes in COPD: a controlled trial. Eur Respir J 2013;42: 982–92.

82. Dernaika TA, Beavin M, Kinasewitz GT. Iloprost improves gas exchange and exercise tolerance in patients with pulmonary hypertension and chronic obstructive pulmonary disease. Respiration 2010; 79(5):377–82.

83. Weissmann N, Lobo B, Pichl A, et al. Stimulation of soluble guanylate cyclase prevents cigarette smoke-induced pulmonary hypertension and emphysema. Am J Respir Crit Care Med 2014; 189(11):1359–73.

84. Vonbank K, Ziesche R, Higenbottam TW, et al. Controlled prospective randomised trial on the effects on pulmonary haemodynamics of the ambulatory long term use of nitric oxide and oxygen in patients with severe COPD. Thorax 2003; 58(4):289–93.

85. Ghofrani HA, Staehler G, Grünig E, et al. Acute effects of riociguat in borderline or manifest pulmonary hypertension associated with chronic obstructive pulmonary disease. Pulm Circ 2015; 5(2):296–304.

86. King TE Jr, Behr J, Brown KK, et al. BUILD-1: a randomized placebo-controlled trial of bosentan in idiopathic pulmonary fibrosis. Am J Respir Crit Care Med 2008;177(1):75–81.

87. King TE Jr, Brown KK, Raghu G, et al. BUILD-3: a randomized, controlled trial of bosentan in idiopathic pulmonary fibrosis. Am J Respir Crit Care Med 2011;184(1):92–9.

88. Raghu G, Behr J, Brown KK, et al, ARTEMIS-IPF Investigators. Treatment of idiopathic pulmonary fibrosis with ambrisentan: a parallel, randomized trial. Ann Intern Med 2013;158(9):641–9.

89. Raghu G, Million-Rousseau R, Morganti A, et al, MUSIC Study Group. Macitentan for the treatment of idiopathic pulmonary fibrosis: the randomised controlled MUSIC trial. Eur Respir J 2013;42(6): 1622–32.

90. Corte TJ, Keir GJ, Dimopoulos K, et al, BPHIT Study Group. Bosentan in pulmonary hypertension associated with fibrotic idiopathic interstitial pneumonia. Am J Respir Crit Care Med 2014;190(2): 208–17.

91. Idiopathic Pulmonary Fibrosis Clinical Research Network, Zisman DA, Schwarz M, Anstrom KJ, et al. A controlled trial of sildenafil in advanced idiopathic pulmonary fibrosis. N Engl J Med 2010; 363(7):620–8.

92. Jackson RM, Glassberg MK, Ramos CF, et al. Sildenafil therapy and exercise tolerance in idiopathic pulmonary fibrosis. Lung 2010;188(2):115–23.

93. Ghofrani HA, Wiedemann R, Rose F, et al. Sildenafil for treatment of lung fibrosis and pulmonary hypertension: a randomised controlled trial. Lancet 2002; 360(9337):895–900.

94. Corte TJ, Gatzoulis MA, Parfitt L, et al. The use of sildenafil to treat pulmonary hypertension associated with interstitial lung disease. Respirology 2010;15(8):1226–32.

95. Han MK, Bach DS, Hagan PG, et al, IPFnet Investigators. Sildenafil preserves exercise capacity in patients with idiopathic pulmonary fibrosis and right-sided ventricular dysfunction. Chest 2013; 143(6):1699–708.

96. Zimmermann GS, von Wulffen W, Huppmann P, et al. Haemodynamic changes in pulmonary hypertension in patients with interstitial lung disease treated with PDE-5 inhibitors. Respirology 2014; 19(5):700–6.

97. Saggar R, Shapiro SS, Ross DJ, et al. Treprostinil to reverse pulmonary hypertension associated with idiopathic pulmonary fibrosis as a bridge to single-lung transplantation. J Heart Lung Transplant 2009;28(9):964–7.

98. Saggar R, Khanna D, Vaidya A, et al. Changes in right heart haemodynamics and echocardiographic function in an advanced phenotype of pulmonary hypertension and right heart dysfunction associated with pulmonary fibrosis. Thorax 2014; 69(2):123–9.

99. Hoeper MM, Halank M, Wilkens H, et al. Riociguat for interstitial lung disease and pulmonary hypertension: a pilot trial. Eur Respir J 2013; 41(4):853–60.

100. Yokoe T, Minoguchi K, Matsuo H, et al. Elevated levels of C-reactive protein and interleukin-6 in patients with obstructive sleep apnea syndrome are decreased by nasal continuous positive airway pressure. Circulation 2003;107(8):1129–34.

101. Bokinsky G, Miller M, Ault K, et al. Spontaneous platelet activation and aggregation during obstructive sleep apnea and its response to therapy with nasal continuous positive airway pressure. A preliminary investigation. Chest 1995;108(3):625–30.

102. Sajkov D, Wang T, Saunders NA, et al. Continuous positive airway pressure treatment improves pulmonary hemodynamics in patients with obstructive sleep apnea. Am J Respir Crit Care Med 2002; 165(2):152–8.

103. Arias MA, García-Río F, Alonso-Fernández A, et al. Pulmonary hypertension in obstructive sleep apnoea: effects of continuous positive airway pressure: a randomized, controlled cross-over study. Eur Heart J 2006;27(9):1106–13.

104. Ip MS, Lam B, Chan LY, et al. Circulating nitric oxide is suppressed in obstructive sleep apnea and is reversed by nasal continuous positive airway pressure. Am J Respir Crit Care Med 2000; 162(6):2166–71.

105. Galiè N, Corris PA, Frost A, et al. Updated treatment algorithm of pulmonary arterial hypertension. J Am Coll Cardiol 2013;62(Suppl 25):D60–72.

106. Taichman DB, Ornelas J, Chung L, et al. Pharmacologic therapy for pulmonary arterial hypertension in adults: CHEST guideline and expert panel report. Chest 2014;146(2):449–75.

107. Rao RS, Singh S, Sharma BB, et al. Sildenafil improves six-minute walk distance in chronic obstructive pulmonary disease: a randomised, double-blind, placebo-controlled trial. Indian J Chest Dis Allied Sci 2011;53(2):81–5.

Group 4 Pulmonary Hypertension
Chronic Thromboembolic Pulmonary Hypertension: Epidemiology, Pathophysiology, and Treatment

Nick H. Kim, MD

KEYWORDS

- Chronic thromboembolic pulmonary hypertension • Chronic thromboembolism
- Pulmonary embolism • Pulmonary thromboendarterectomy • Pulmonary endarterectomy
- Riociguat • Balloon pulmonary angioplasty

KEY POINTS

- Pulmonary embolism history can be absent in chronic thromboembolic pulmonary hypertension (CTEPH).
- Negative computed tomography pulmonary angiogram does not rule out CTEPH.
- Pulmonary thromboendarterectomy remains the treatment of choice for CTEPH.
- Operability assessment should be performed by an experienced CTEPH team.

The first successful pulmonary thromboendarterectomy (PTE) for the treatment of chronic thromboembolic pulmonary hypertension (CTEPH) was reported nearly 20 years before the introduction of both heart-lung transplantation and intravenous epoprostenol for the treatment of pulmonary arterial hypertension (PAH).[1–3] Fast forward another 30 years, and much has evolved in our understanding and treatment of pulmonary hypertension (PH), and with that, so has our approach to the diagnosis and management of patients with CTEPH.

EPIDEMIOLOGY

CTEPH is a complication of pulmonary embolism.[4,5] Although the true incidence of CTEPH following acute pulmonary embolism remains unknown, reports have ranged widely from 0.4% to 9.1%.[4,6–10] The variability of the incidence reports may reflect differences in patient selection and methodology across these reports. Whether these rates represent true incidence of CTEPH after acute pulmonary embolism, or combination of incident and prevalent cases remains speculative. For example, in the series of Pengo and colleagues,[4] no additional CTEPH was detected beyond 2 years from the initial acute pulmonary embolism, and one of the cases reportedly developed near-systemic PH within just 5 months from the acute event. The characteristics of these cases arguably raise concerns that the series of Pengo and colleagues[4] may not be solely an incident series of CTEPH occurring after acute pulmonary embolism, but rather one that unintentionally included both incident and previously unrecognized CTEPH cases.

Additional efforts are currently under way to prospectively capture incident cases of CTEPH by screening after acute, first-time pulmonary

Disclosures: Consultancy/Speakers Bureau: Actelion, Bayer; Board Member: CTEPH.com.
Division of Pulmonary and Critical Care Medicine, University of California, San Diego, 9300 Campus Point Drive, MC 7381, La Jolla, CA 92037, USA
E-mail address: h33kim@ucsd.edu

Cardiol Clin 34 (2016) 435–441
http://dx.doi.org/10.1016/j.ccl.2016.04.011
0733-8651/16/$ – see front matter

cardiology.theclinics.com

embolism cases to better assess the true incidence of CTEPH. Nevertheless, any measurement or estimate of CTEPH incidence after acute pulmonary embolism may underestimate the overall burden of CTEPH because as many as 25% to 30% of patients with CTEPH are diagnosed without a prior clinical history of pulmonary embolism, and nearly half of these patients may not have a history of deep venous thrombosis.[11,12] Therefore, a key take-home point when evaluating patients presenting with PH is that the lack of a venous thromboembolism history should not exclude CTEPH as a possibility.

Table 1 shows epidemiologic data used to estimate the incidence of CTEPH to better appreciate the scope of CTEPH in the United States.[13] The calculations shown are based on the CTEPH incidence rate reported from Klok and colleagues.[7] This study included the largest pulmonary embolism series (866 consecutive cases) screened for CTEPH following standard diagnostic guidelines including right heart catheterization. Even using this lower range of the reported incidence rates after pulmonary embolism, approximately 3400 cases of CTEPH in the United States might be expected each year. Combined with the approximately 30% of CTEPH cases operated without a history of prior pulmonary embolism, the overall estimate of new CTEPH cases diagnosed in the United States each year jumps to nearly 5000 new CTEPH cases per year.

An important question today then is: Where are these patients with CTEPH and how are they being treated? Although precise data on the number of PTE surgeries performed in the United States is not known, estimated 300 to 400 PTEs are being performed in the United States per year today. However, based on estimates from Table 1, this represents fewer than 8% of incident CTEPH cases being operated annually. Even when accounting for the limitations of such extrapolated estimates, there appears to be a large discrepancy between number of potentially surgically treatable cases and surgically treated volume. Table 2 lists the plausible reasons behind this large gap. In addition to possibly inaccurate incidence rates, cases of CTEPH may not be properly diagnosed, and if diagnosed, may not be referred for surgical treatment as recommended consistently by best practice guidelines.[14,15]

One particular diagnostic pitfall in CTEPH is the failure to obtain a lung ventilation perfusion (VQ) scan to screen for CTEPH during the workup of PH.[16] Computed tomography (CT) pulmonary angiography is often (erroneously) used in place of the VQ scan. Unfortunately, CT pulmonary angiography lacks adequate sensitivity to detect

Table 1
Estimated annual incidence of CTEPH in the United States

	Estimates
PE cases per year[13]	600,000
Incidence of CTEPH after PE[7]	0.57%
CTEPH cases after PE per year	3420
Additional 30% of CTEPH cases per year without prior pulmonary embolism	1466
Total overall CTEPH cases estimated per year	4886

Abbreviations: CTEPH, chronic thromboembolic pulmonary hypertension; PE, pulmonary embolism.

Table 2
Potential explanations for the gap between estimated CTEPH incidence from Table 1, and the relatively small number of PTE cases performed in the United States

Explanation	Result
Assumptions are incorrect	
Examples: • PE estimate may not be accurate • Some PE cases may have had CTEPH already (ie, not incident PE) • CTEPH true incidence may be lower	Error in true incidence of CTEPH
CTEPH is not being diagnosed	
Examples: • Failure to recognize/ diagnose CTEPH • CTEPH Incorrectly diagnosed as PAH • CTEPH Incorrectly diagnosed as recurrent pulmonary embolism	CTEPH is underestimated
Under referral for CTEPH evaluation/treatment	
Examples: • Providers not aware of PTE surgery or have limited access • Operability is being decided locally • Medical treatment is elected instead of PTE	CTEPH is underestimated

Abbreviations: CTEPH, chronic thromboembolic pulmonary hypertension; PAH, pulmonary arterial hypertension; PE, pulmonary embolism; PTE, pulmonary thromboendarterectomy.

CTEPH detection, and therefore cannot reliably rule out CTEPH, whereas the VQ scan is more sensitive.[14,17]

Fig. 1 show an example of an abnormal VQ scan and the corresponding CT angiogram done in the same patient, which was read as "negative for pulmonary embolism." The CT reading is correct; there is no pulmonary embolism. However, there is evidence of CTEPH with eccentric lining material in the left descending pulmonary artery, segmental webs, bronchial collaterals, and right ventricular hypertrophy (not shown on this image). These sometimes-subtle defects suggestive of CTEPH on CT can be overlooked leading to a false negative study. So with a negative pulmonary embolism report, this CT pulmonary angiogram may contribute to eventual misdiagnosis of PAH when the patient in actuality has CTEPH. On a VQ scan, pulmonary embolism and CTEPH appear identical in revealing perfusion defects – and hence bypassing the need for additional training for the radiologist or reviewer. But for CT pulmonary angiograms, acute pulmonary embolism and chronic thromboembolic disease of CTEPH appear quite differently despite sharing similar perfusion defects on VQ scan.

PATHOPHYSIOLOGY OF CHRONIC THROMBOEMBOLIC PULMONARY HYPERTENSION

Although linked with pulmonary embolism, the pathophysiologic development of CTEPH extends beyond thrombosis. In one large registry, more than two-thirds of patients with CTEPH had no identifiable coagulopathy contributing to susceptibility.[11] Of the numerous types of thrombophilia, lupus anticoagulant and antiphospholipid syndrome have been associated with CTEPH in only 10% to 20% of reported cases. Therefore, the

efforts to understand the pathogenesis of CTEPH have focused beyond thrombosis.

Multiple medical comorbidities are more commonly present in patients with CTEPH than those with PAH.[18] These conditions may offer clues to potential pathogenic mechanisms contributing to the development of CTEPH. In a large series comparing CTEPH and PAH populations, the presence of ventriculoatrial (VA) shunt, infected pacemaker, or history of splenectomy had the highest odds ratios for the development of CTEPH, higher even than a history of recurrent venous thromboembolism. Although the precise link between these associated comorbidities and CTEPH is not known, inflammation and infection have been hypothesized as contributors for the development of CTEPH in these at-risk populations.[5,19]

In a report from Bonderman and colleagues,[19] of 7 consecutively operated VA shunt associated CTEPH cases, 6 had staphylococcal DNA isolated from the endarterectomized tissue. They also found that in a murine model of inferior vena cava thrombosis that staphylococcal infection delayed resolution of thrombi and decreased expression of macrophages, cells that are vital to thrombus resolution. More recently, a group from Belgium studied 52 operated CTEPH cases and reported associated abnormalities in neovascularization.[20] The endarterectomized specimens were also noted to have abundance of macrophages, lymphocytes, and neutrophils within the chronic thromboembolic material. With elevations in numerous proinflammatory markers and cytokines in CTEPH compared with controls, a compelling case can be made for active inflammatory process contributing to the development of CTEPH. Furthermore, Zabini and colleagues[21] reported that both interferon gamma-induced protein 10 (IP-10) and interleukin-6 levels were positively and negatively correlated with hemodynamics and exercise capacity, respectively, in

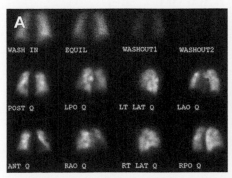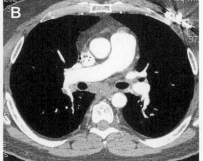

Fig. 1. (*A*) VQ scan showing multiple segmental and subsegmental perfusion defects. (*B*) CT pulmonary angiogram revealed no pulmonary embolism, but on closer review demonstrates signs of chronic disease.

CTEPH. IP-10 is associated with fibroblast migration and activation, which may be important in the development of chronic intimal fibrosis of the pulmonary arteries in CTEPH. Together with prior reports of abnormal fibrinolysis in some cases of CTEPH, the research focus has once again been shifted away from simply a problem of thrombosis, to a failure to adequately clear the thrombotic insult, influenced potentially by multiple factors including an inflammatory response, infection, and fibrin resistance.[5,22]

The role of small vessel abnormalities in the lungs of patients with CTEPH has received a recent major update from the work of Dorfmuller and colleagues.[23] In their histopathologic report of 17 CTEPH cases with either distal, inoperable CTEPH, or residual PH after pulmonary endarterectomy, the scope of small vessel involvement of CTEPH was found to extend beyond the precapillary small arteries. They found significant disease in the pulmonary venous and capillary systems, similar to that seen in pulmonary veno-occlusive disease and pulmonary capillary hemangiomatosis, respectively, as well as impressive systemic-pulmonary anastomoses and hypertrophied bronchial collaterals. These observations are important reminders that CTEPH is not just chronic thrombus with varying degrees of precapillary changes similar to idiopathic PAH, but rather, a more complex disease with heterogeneous and less predictable involvement of the entire pulmonary circulation and associated collateral vasculature.

As the microvasculature in CTEPH appears to be different from PAH, it is not a stretch to surmise that the RV in CTEPH may also be different compared with that of other forms of PH. The primary location of vascular resistance in the pulmonary circulation appears to affect the RV afterload differently. In a canine model of PH, Pagnamenta and colleagues[24] reported differences in RV afterload between proximal versus distal obstruction of the pulmonary arterial bed. Using models of proximal pulmonary artery ensnarement and distal micro-embolization to differentiate proximal versus distal pulmonary vascular obstruction, the investigators noted that for similar degrees of PH, the RV time constant was lower and the RV afterload higher for the proximal obstruction model. MacKenzie and colleagues[25] also observed differences between CTEPH and PAH. For a given mean pulmonary arterial pressure, the RV time constant was significantly shorter in CTEPH compared with PAH. For similar degree of PH, the investigators concluded that the RV in CTEPH has greater burden of work than in PAH. This may explain the observations reported by Giusca and colleagues[26] when comparing echocardiograms from varying causes of PH. In this report, patients with CTEPH exhibited the lowest tricuspid annular plane systolic excursion (indicating lower RV contractility) and the smallest RV fractional area change compared with both patients with PAH and patients with Eisenmenger syndrome. Taken together, these findings suggest that the RV in CTEPH may not adapt as well to the type of afterload posed by CTEPH (proximal disease component) as other forms of PH. This may have implications on RV recovery and targeting of therapies for CTEPH. For example, the RV in CTEPH may have differential recovery or response depending on whether we relieve the proximal mechanical disease versus the microvascular component.

The pathophysiology of CTEPH therefore is multifaceted and goes beyond thrombosis (**Fig. 2**). In reviewing the treatment of CTEPH, it is helpful to consider these various components

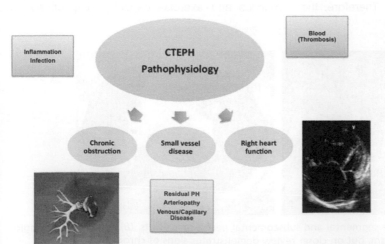

Fig. 2. Pathophysiology of CTEPH goes beyond thrombosis.

Box 1
Steps to take after chronic thromboembolic pulmonary hypertension (CTEPH) diagnosis

1. Chronic anticoagulation therapy
2. Refer for pulmonary thromboendarterectomy (PTE) consideration[a]
3. If deemed not to be a surgical candidate, consider the following options
4a. Medical therapy for inoperable disease
4b. Consider referral for balloon pulmonary angioplasty option
4c. Consider second opinion for possible PTE
5. If not responding/candidate for any above treatments, refer for lung transplantation

[a] Can be initially a remote review by a CTEPH team of pertinent records and images.

---

to better understand treatment priorities as well as some limitations, and potentially future opportunities, of our current approach.

TREATMENT

The first steps after CTEPH diagnosis should always include chronic anticoagulation and consideration of PTE surgery.[14] **Box 1** outlines a simplified stepwise approach to every case of newly diagnosed CTEPH. The optimal method of chronic anticoagulation has not been studied. Despite the availability of newer oral anticoagulant therapies, it is unknown if these agents are safe and effective in the treatment or maintenance

phase of CTEPH.[27] In addition to chronic anticoagulation, all patients should be referred to a CTEPH team for operability assessment.[14] The determination of operability combines objective data, such as patient factors, hemodynamics, and imaging, but critically also hinges on surgical or center experience (**Fig. 3**). Such subjectivity needs to be considered when interpreting treatment decisions. For example, an inexperienced reviewer turning a case down for surgery is possibly depriving that patient of a potentially curative surgical intervention.

PTE remains the principal treatment of choice for CTEPH. The surgery is not an embolectomy or thrombectomy, but a true endarterectomy, involving stripping of the inner layer of both pulmonary arteries to restore distal blood flow and relieve the PH. Following successful PTE, compliance to chronic anticoagulation therapy should obviate the need for second surgery. For patients with CTEPH deemed inoperable due to technically distal (unreachable) disease, or for patients with residual PH following PTE, riociguat is the only approved medical therapy.[28] It should be noted that riociguat (or any other off-label PAH-targeted medical therapy) should not be prescribed for patients with operable CTEPH. The risks and benefits of these treatments in CTEPH have not been adequately tested and such patients should undergo PTE surgery without delay.[29]

In addition to riociguat, select patients with inoperable CTEPH may be candidates for percutaneous transluminal pulmonary angioplasty, also referred to as balloon pulmonary angioplasty (BPA).[14,30,31] Although recent refinements have made this procedure a safer and viable alternative

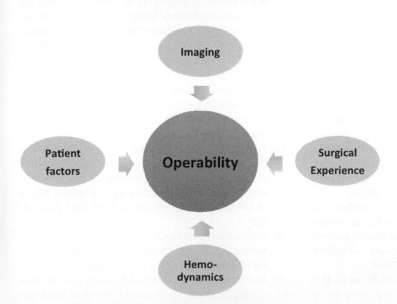

Fig. 3. CTEPH operability assessment requires consideration of multiple and both objective and subjective factors.

when conventional therapy is not available, patient selection and treatment need to be performed by experienced specialists, much like the case with PTE surgery. Significant complications, including procedure-related deaths, have been reported with an overall complication rates as high as 60%.[30,32] Finally, the precise role of BPA in the treatment algorithm of CTEPH and its relation to PTE and medical therapy remain unclear and in need of clarification.

SUMMARY

CTEPH is a unique and important type of PH, one that may dramatically respond to timely and appropriate intervention. There is a growing awareness worldwide of CTEPH and its pathogenesis is being better defined, but more work is needed in both awareness and pathogenesis. Treatment options have expanded to include targeted, effective medical therapy for eligible patients, as well as an emerging catheter-based interventions. Due to the many nuances of CTEPH, all such treatment decisions should be coordinated with an experienced CTEPH team to provide the best and most appropriate treatment for the individual patient.

REFERENCES

1. Houk VN, Hufnagel CA, McClenathan JE, et al. Chronic thrombotic obstruction of major pulmonary arteries. Report of a case successfully treated by thromboendarterectomy, and a review of the literature. Am J Med 1963;35:269–82.
2. Reitz BA, Wallwork JL, Hunt SA, et al. Heart-lung transplantation: successful therapy for patients with pulmonary vascular disease. N Engl J Med 1982; 306:557–64.
3. Rubin LJ, Groves B, Reeves JT, et al. Prostacyclin-induced acute pulmonary vasodilation in primary pulmonary hypertension. Circulation 1982;66:334–8.
4. Pengo V, Lensing AW, Prins MH, et al. Incidence of chronic thromboembolic pulmonary hypertension after pulmonary embolism. N Engl J Med 2004;350: 2257–64.
5. Lang IM, Pesavento R, Bonderman D, et al. Risk factors and basic mechanisms of chronic thromboembolic pulmonary hypertension: a current understanding. Eur Respir J 2013;41:462–8.
6. Poli D, Grifoni E, Antonucci E, et al. Incidence of recurrent venous thromboembolism and of chronic thromboembolic pulmonary hypertension in patients after a first episode of pulmonary embolism. J Thromb Thrombolysis 2010;30:294–9.
7. Klok FA, van Kralingen KW, van Dijk AP, et al. Prospective cardiopulmonary screening program to detect chronic thromboembolic pulmonary hypertension in patients after acute pulmonary embolism. Haematologica 2010;95:970–5.
8. Yang S, Yang Y, Zhai Z, et al. Incidence and risk factors of chronic thromboembolic pulmonary hypertension in patients after acute pulmonary embolism. J Thorac Dis 2015;7:1927–38.
9. Guérin L, Couturaud F, Parent F, et al. Prevalence of chronic thromboembolic pulmonary hypertension after acute pulmonary embolism. Prevalence of CTEPH after pulmonary embolism. Thromb Haemost 2014;112:598–605.
10. Marti D, Gomez V, Escobar C, et al. Incidence of symptomatic and asymptomatic chronic thromboembolic pulmonary hypertension. Arch Bronconeumol 2010;46:628–33.
11. Pepke-Zaba J, Delcroix M, Lang I, et al. Chronic thromboembolic pulmonary hypertension (CTEPH): results from an international prospective registry. Circulation 2011;124:1973–81.
12. Lang IM, Madani M. Update on chronic thromboembolic pulmonary hypertension. Circulation 2014;130: 508–18.
13. Hirsh J, Hoak J. Management of deep vein thrombosis and pulmonary embolism. A statement for healthcare professionals from the council on thrombosis (in consultation with the council on cardiovascular radiology), American Heart Association. Circulation 1996;93:2212–45.
14. Kim NH, Delcroix M, Jenkins DP, et al. Chronic thromboembolic pulmonary hypertension. J Am Coll Cardiol 2013;62:D92–9.
15. Galiè N, Humbert M, Vachiery JL, et al. 2015 ESC/ERS guidelines for the diagnosis and treatment of pulmonary hypertension: the joint task force for the diagnosis and treatment of pulmonary hypertension of the European Society of Cardiology (ESC) and the European Respiratory Society (ERS): endorsed by: Association for European Paediatric and Congenital Cardiology (AEPC), International Society for Heart and Lung Transplantation (ISHLT). Eur Respir J 2015;46:903–75.
16. McLaughlin VV, Langer A, Tan M, et al. Contemporary trends in the diagnosis and management of pulmonary arterial hypertension: an initiative to close the care gap. Chest 2013;143:324–32.
17. Tunariu N, Gibbs SJ, Win Z, et al. Ventilation-perfusion scintigraphy is more sensitive than multidetector CTPA in detecting chronic thromboembolic pulmonary disease as a treatable cause of pulmonary hypertension. J Nucl Med 2007;48: 680–4.
18. Bonderman D, Wilkens H, Wakounig S, et al. Risk factors for chronic thromboembolic pulmonary hypertension. Eur Respir J 2009;33:325–31.
19. Bonderman D, Jakowitsch J, Redwan B, et al. Role of staphylococci in misguided thrombus resolution

...onic thromboembolic pulmonary hypertension. Arterioscler Thromb Vasc Biol 2008;28:678–84.

20. Quarck R, Wynants M, Verbeken E, et al. Contribution of inflammation and impaired angiogenesis to the pathobiology of chronic thromboembolic pulmonary hypertension. Eur Respir J 2015;46:431–43.

21. Zabini D, Heinemann A, Foris V, et al. Comprehensive analysis of inflammatory markers in chronic thromboembolic pulmonary hypertension patients. Eur Respir J 2013;44:951–62.

22. Morris TA, March JJ, Chiles PG, et al. High prevalence of dysfibrinogenemia among patients with chronic thromboembolic pulmonary hypertension. Blood 2009;114:1929–36.

23. Dorfmuller P, Gunther S, Ghigna MR, et al. Microvascular disease in chronic thromboembolic pulmonary hypertension: a role for pulmonary veins and systemic vasculature. Eur Respir J 2014;44:1275–88.

24. Pagnamenta A, Vanderpool R, Brimioulle S, et al. Proximal pulmonary arterial obstruction decreases the time constant of the pulmonary circulation and increases right ventricular afterload. J Appl Physiol (1985) 2013;114:1586–92.

25. MacKenzie Ross RV, Toshner MR, Soon E, et al. Decreased time constant of the pulmonary circulation in chronic thromboembolic pulmonary hypertension. Am J Physiol Heart Circ Physiol 2013;305: H259–64.

26. Giusca S, Popa E, Amzulescu MS, et al. ...tricular remodeling in pulmonary hy... dependent on etiology? An echocardi... study. Echocardiography 2016;33(4):546–54.

27. Hinojar R, Jimenez-Natcher JJ, Fernandez-Go... et al. New oral anticoagulants: a practical guide... physicians. Eur Heart J Cardiovasc Pharmacoth... 2015;1:134–45.

28. Ghofrani HA, D'Armini AM, Grimminger F, et al. Riociguat for the treatment of chronic thromboembolic pulmonary hypertension. N Engl J Med 2013;369: 319–29.

29. Jensen KW, Kerr KM, Fedullo PF, et al. Pulmonary hypertensive medical therapy in chronic thromboembolic pulmonary hypertension before pulmonary endarterectomy. Circulation 2009;120:1248–54.

30. Mizoguchi H, Ogawa A, Munemasa M, et al. Refined balloon pulmonary angioplasty for inoperable patients with chronic thromboembolic pulmonary hypertension. Circ Cardiovasc Interv 2012;5:748–55.

31. Inami T, Kataoka M, Ishiguro H, et al. Percutaneous transluminal pulmonary angioplasty for chronic thromboembolic pulmonary hypertension with severe right heart failure. Am J Respir Crit Care Med 2014;189:1437–9.

32. Feinstein JA, Goldhaber SZ, Lock JE, et al. Balloon pulmonary angioplasty for treatment of chronic thromboembolic pulmonary hypertension. Circulation 2001;103:10–3.

Group 5 Pulmonary Hypertension
The Orphan's Orphan Disease

Sara Kalantari, MD[a],
Mardi Gomberg-Maitland, MD, MSc[a,b],*

KEYWORDS

- Pulmonary hypertension • Multifactorial • Chronic thromboembolic pulmonary hypertension

KEY POINTS

- Group 5 pulmonary hypertension (PH) contains a variety of diseases that can be subcategorized into hematologic disorders, systemic disorders, and metabolic disorders.
- The true prevalence of PH defined using the gold standard of right heart catheterization (RHC) is unknown in most of these disorders and the cause is multifactorial.
- Evidence-based pathogenesis and management are mostly guided by case reports or small case series. In general, treatment of group 5 PH is directed toward treating the underlying condition, with consideration of pulmonary arterial hypertension (PAH) therapies based on clinical characteristics on a case-by-case basis.

INTRODUCTION

PH is a complex disorder with multiple etiologies; as such, the World Health Organization classification system divides PH patients into 5 groups based on the underlying cause and mechanism. This classification system is designed to help organize diagnostic evaluations and direct treatment. Group 5 PH is an important heterogeneous group of diseases that encompass PH secondary to multifactorial mechanisms. For many of the diseases, the true incidence, etiology, and treatment remain uncertain.[1,2] Increased vascular resistance can occur secondary to hypoxic vasoconstriction, inflammation, proliferative arteriopathy shunting, chronic anemia, veno-occlusive disease, left ventricular dysfunction, and valvular heart disease. This article reviews the epidemiology, pathogenesis, and management of many of the various group 5 PH disease states.

GROUP 5.1: HEMATOLOGIC DISORDERS
Chronic Myeloproliferative Diseases

Chronic myeloproliferative diseases (CMPDs) are a heterogeneous group of diseases with different genetic bases. Myeloproliferative diseases, including polycythemia vera, essential thrombocythemia, and primary myelofibrosis, have been associated with PH.

Disclosures: The University of Chicago receives research grant support from Actelion, Bayer, Gilead, Novartis, Medtronic, Lung Biotechnology, and Reata for Dr M. Gomberg-Maitland to be a principal investigator on research grants. Dr M. Gomberg-Maitland has served as a consultant for Actelion, Bayer, Bellerophon, GeNO, Gilead, Medtronic, and United Therapeutics as a member of steering committees and DSMB/event committees. She has received honoraria for CME from Medscape and ABComm. Dr M. Gomberg-Maitland is a member of the PCORI Advisory Panel on Rare Diseases. Dr S. Kalantari has no conflicts of interest.
 a Section of Cardiology, Department of Medicine, University of Chicago Medical Center, 5841 South Maryland Avenue, MC 5403, Chicago, IL 60637, USA; b Pulmonary Hypertension Program, Cardiovascular Division, University of Chicago Medical Center, 5841 South Maryland Avenue, MC 5403, Chicago, IL 60637, USA
* Corresponding author. Pulmonary Hypertension Program, Cardiovascular Division, University of Chicago Medical Center, 5841 South Maryland Avenue, MC 5403, Chicago, IL 60637.
E-mail address: mgomberg@bsd.uchicago.edu

Cardiol Clin 34 (2016) 443–449
http://dx.doi.org/10.1016/j.ccl.2016.04.004

Prevalence/etiology

The true prevalence of PH in CMPD using hemodynamic criteria by RHC is unknown. Small case reports have reported a prevalence of PH (as defined by estimated RV systolic pressure ≥35 using transthoracic echo) in 36% to 48% of cohorts.[3,4] The etiology of PH in myeloproliferative diseases is multifactorial and has been associated with chronic thromboembolic PH (CTEPH), vascular remodeling, pulmonary veno-occlusive disease, tumor microembolism, and drug-induced PH.[5] CMPDs, in particular polycythemia vera and essential thrombocythemia, are characterized by a thrombophilic state, which may lead to arterial and venous thrombosis.[6] CMPD patients treated with the tyrosine kinase inhibitor dasatinib have also developed PAH.[7]

Treatment

There is no known effective treatment of PH associated with CMPDs. There is minimal evidence to support the use of cytoreductive (hydroxyurea and antiplatelet agents) therapy, which is effective in treating risk of thrombosis and vascular events in CMPD and may be effective in treating CMPD-PH.[5,8] There are few data to guide the role of pulmonary vasodilators in patients with CMPD-associated PH.[9,10] Standard-of-care clinical follow-up, however, with biomarkers, imaging, and cardiac catheterization should be done if these therapeutics are used.

Postsplenectomy

Incidence

Splenectomy may be a risk factor for PH.[11] After splenectomy, thrombotic and thromboembolic complications can occur. One retrospective study found a 10% incidence of pulmonary thromboembolic disease in 150 patients postsplenectomy.[12] Splenectomy has been associated with chronic thromboembolic pulmonary hypertension (CTEPH) as well as idiopathic PAH.[11,13]

Etiology

The etiology of thromboembolism postsplenectomy is not well understood. Splenectomy is associated with thrombocytosis; however, this has not been shown associated with increased thromboembolic risk.[14] There are minimal data on the presence of a hypercoagulable state postsplenectomy. The loss of the spleen's filtering function allows abnormal red cells to remain in the peripheral circulation after splenectomy, which may lead to facilitation of the coagulation process, which has been demonstrated in vivo.[15]

Treatment

Patients who present with PAH postsplenectomy without evidence of CTEPH may be treated with PAH-specific therapies and follow PAH group 1 guidelines.[4]

If possible, splenectomy-associated proximal CTEPH should be treated with surgical pulmonary endarterectomy.[16] If pulmonary endarterectomy is not possible due to anatomic distribution of the disease or comorbidities, then medical treatment consists of anticoagulation and diuretics with consideration of specific PAH therapy or lung transplantation. Two randomized placebo-controlled studies, one with bosentan, an endothelin receptor antagonist, and the other with riociguat, a guanylate cyclase stimulator, with inoperable or persistent CTEPH after thromboendarterectomy, improved exercise capacity and hemodynamics.[17,18]

The role for anticoagulation prophylactics to prevent CTEPH after splenectomy is unclear. A case-based approach evaluating each patient's risk of thromboembolic disease is likely warranted. Patients with asplenia in whom PH is suspected should undergo thorough assessment for thromboembolic disease with ventilation perfusion scanning and CT angiography.

Chronic Hemolytic Anemia – Sickle Cell Disease

Incidence

PH associated with chronic hemolytic anemia secondary to hemoglobinopathies recently moved from group 1 PAH to group 5.[1] This switch occurred due to its mixed etiology PH presentations. Sickle cell anemia results from a genetic mutation leading to the production of hemoglobin S, which is less soluble when deoxygenated than the normal hemoglobin molecule, hemoglobin A.[19] Deoxygenated hemoglobin S polymerizes and aggregates, leading to microvascular occlusion and chronic hemolytic anemia. Three recent studies using RHC data to evaluate the incidence of PH among patients with sickle cell disease (SCD) found a prevalence of 6% to 10.5% and that the presence of PH was a major risk factor for death.[20–22]

Etiology

RHC data has revealed both precapillary PH as well as pulmonary venous hypertension secondary to left ventricular dysfunction in patients with SCD and PH.[20–22] PH has not been associated with the number of vasoocclusive episodes or acute chest syndrome, only with abnormalities in hemolytic anemia markers. Screening studies of patients with SCD have shown an association between the degree of hemolysis and the development of PH.[22] Some investigators propose that plasma-free hemoglobin that is released during hemolysis leads to decreased nitric oxide bioavailability, potentially mechanistically linking hemolysis with PH.[23] The high cardiac output state secondary to chronic hemolysis and resultant anemia might also lead to an increased pulmonary artery pressure. Many adult SCD patients have mildly restrictive abnormalities on pulmonary function testing; however, these abnormalities are rarely severe enough to lead to group 3 PH.[24] Among SCD-PH patients, CTEPH has been identified in approximately 5%.[25]

Treatment

There are few data to guide the management for patients with chronic hemolytic anemia and PH. A reasonable approach is to attempt to treat the underlying disease to minimize hemolysis and associated cardiopulmonary conditions. Treatment with PAH therapies have not been successful. The Walk-PHaSST study (sildenafil therapy for PH and SCD) was a multicenter National Institutes of Health double-blind placebo-controlled trial of sildenafil in patients with SCD that was stopped early because of a higher incidence of serious adverse events in the sildenafil arm. This was primarily caused by increased hospitalization for vasoocclusive pain crisis with no suggestion of improvement.[26] The ASSET-1 and ASSET-2 studies aimed to assess the efficacy and safety of bosentan therapy in patients with SCD and PAH; however, the studies were terminated due to lack of overt efficacy, slow site activation, and withdrawal of sponsor support.[27] Although epoprostenol acutely improves hemodynamics in these patients, there have been no studies of chronic long-term therapy.[28] Despite anecdotal experience of benefit with oral and continuous infusion in a select group of SCD patients, PAH therapy is not recommended for routine use in PH-SCD patients.[4]

Chronic Hemolytic Anemia – Thalassemia

Thalassemia is caused by a spectrum of diseases with reduced or absent production of 1 or more α-globin or β-globin chains, leading to hemolytic anemia and ineffective erythropoiesis. Small studies using echocardiographically defined PH found a prevalence of 60% in cases with thalassemia intermedia and 75% in patients with thalassemia major; however, the true prevalence is unknown. The etiology is unknown but likely multifactorial with contributions from hemolysis, hypoxia, hypercoagulability, and high CO.[29,30] As part of the National Institutes of Health Thalassemia

Clinical Research Network, patients with β-thalassemia and echocardiographically defined PH received sildenafil. Although no safety concerns arose and the tricuspid regurgitant jet velocity decreased, there was no statistical significant improvement in functional class or the 6-minute walk distance test.[31] No large-scale randomized studies have been done, with only cardiac catheterization reports demonstrating exercise capacity and hemodynamic improvements with PAH therapies.[32]

GROUP 5.2: SYSTEMIC DISORDERS
Sarcoid-Associated Pulmonary Hypertension

Incidence

The incidence of sarcoidosis and PH has been estimated to be between 5% and 28% but may be as high as 75% in patients awaiting lung transplantation.[33,34] In these studies, the presence of PH was associated with increased morbidity and mortality. The presence of lung disease, a low diffusing capacity, and hypoxia on 6-minute walk test are strong risk factors for the presence of PH.[35] Symptoms are often nonspecific and may overlap with symptoms associated with their lung disease leading to underdiagnosis. There is a high variability in presentation: patients may present with dyspnea, right-sided heart failure symptoms, syncope, or sudden death.[4,36]

Etiology

The etiology of sarcoid-associated pulmonary hypertension (SAPH) is often multifactorial. Mechanisms include fibrotic lung involvement leading to the destruction of the pulmonary vascular bed, extrinsic compression of pulmonary vessels leading to altered vascular mechanics, intrinsic vasculopathy, vasculitis involving the pulmonary vasculature, pulmonary veno-occlusion, porto-PH, and left ventricular dysfunction.[37] One series of 40 autopsy studies revealed that granulomatous vascular involvement was common in all levels from large pulmonary arteries to venules. This led to destruction of elastic fibers with eventual replacement of fibrous tissue in the vessel walls.[38] This type of active inflammation and fibrosis led to occlusive vasculopathy. The granulomatous vascular involvement occurs heterogeneously but more frequently involves the venules, leading to a phenotype similar to pulmonary veno-occlusive disease.[38]

Myocardial granulomatous inflammation and fibrosis involvement can lead to systolic and diastolic dysfunction as well as mitral valve pathology. Overall survival in patients with SAPH secondary to left ventricular dysfunction is better than in patients with SAPH secondary to other causes.[39]

Treatment

SAPH studies with PAH-specific therapies are not conclusive.[40,41] One small case series suggested a favorable hemodynamic response to short-term treatment with inhaled nitric oxide[40] A recent case series of 26 patients with SAPH, of whom 13 received treatment with long-term IV or subcutaneous prostacyclin therapy, revealed that prostacyclin therapy was well tolerated with signs of both hemodynamic (RHC: cardiac output and pulmonary vascular resistance) and clinical improvement.[42] Vasodilatory testing is not recommended to determine if calcium channel blockers will be a successful monotherapy but may be used to help differentiate the different etiologies for PH (PH groups 1, 2, and 3).[4] Because the development of SAPH can be caused by multiple different pathophysiologic mechanisms, it is likely that the degree of vasoresponsiveness may be related to the underlying pathology. Those patients with extensive fibrosis and destruction of pulmonary vessels may be less responsive to vasodilator therapy. More investigational studies are needed to evaluate vasodilator therapies.

Pulmonary Langerhans Cell Histiocytosis–Pulmonary Hypertension

Pulmonary Langerhans cell histiocytosis (PLCH) is a rare disease characterized by lung nodules and cystic lesions that is strongly associated with cigarette smoking. The true incidence of PH is unknown, but studies suggest that it is common and associated with high morbidity and mortality.[43,44] The etiology of PLCH-PH is unknown, but some studies suggest pulmonary vascular pathology leading to precapillary PH. Up to one-third of patients have a positive vasodilator response, and a French registry suggested a trend toward improved survival with PAH therapy; however, there are few data to support specific treatment of PLCH-PH.[43,44]

GROUP 5.3: METABOLIC DISORDERS
Thyroid Disease

Incidence

PH patients have a high prevalence of thyroid disease[45,46] of approximately 20%.[47] One small observational study of 63 patients with PAH found that approximately half of these patients had concomitant autoimmune thyroid disease.[46] One case report noted a prevalence of 6.7% of thyroid-stimulating immunoglobulin-negative thyrotoxicosis in patients with preexisting PAH being treated with epoprostenol.[48]

Etiology

A common autoimmune process may be the underlying pathology for PH and associated thyroid disease. Patients with PAH have an increased prevalence of both antithyroglobulin and antithyroperoxidase antibodies.[46] Left ventricular dysfunction can also be seen in the setting of thyroid disease and may contribute to the development of PH.[45] Thyroid disease may also have a direct effect on pulmonary vasculature. Possible mechanisms include enhanced catecholamine sensitivity, increased metabolism of intrinsic pulmonary vasodilators, and decreased metabolism of vasoconstrictors.[49] A high cardiac output state in the setting of hyperthyroidism may also contribute to the development of PH.

Treatment

The development of thyroid disease can lead to arrhythmias and worsening right heart failure and requires immediate attention. Case reports support that the treatment of hyperthyroidism by antithyroid medications, radioactive iodine, surgery or a combination is associated with decreased pulmonary artery pressure.[47] The potential effects of calcium blockers, endothelin receptor blockers, phosphodiesterase 5 inhibitors, or prostacyclins in patients with PH and thyroid disease are not known.

Glycogen Storage Disease–Pulmonary Hypertension

Glycogen storage diseases (GSDs) are characterized by enzymatic deficiencies that lead to defective glycogen synthesis or breakdown leading to abnormal glycogen deposition primarily in muscles and liver. There are 11 different types of GSD, and PH has primarily been described in GSD type 1 (von Gierke disease). The incidence of PH in GSD type 1 is unknown, but it is associated with increased morbidity and mortality and is usually diagnosed in patients in their second or third decade.[50] The etiology of GSD-PH is unknown; however, it has been postulated that abnormalities in serotonin metabolism may contribute.[50] There is no known treatment of GSD-PH.

Gaucher Disease–Pulmonary Hypertension

Gaucher disease (GD) is the most common lysosomal storage disease and is a genetic disorder caused by a deficiency of the enzyme glucocerebrosidase that leads to glucocerebroside accumulation in macrophages and subsequent organ infiltration. Type 1 GD has been associated with

PH and has been described as occurring in up to 30% of untreated patients using echocardiographically defined PH. The etiology is unknown but may be secondary to direct pulmonary capillary infiltration as well as bone marrow microemboli leading to vasculopathy.[51] Splenectomy (described previously) has also been postulated as contributing to the development of PH.[52] GD-PH usually improves with enzyme replacement therapy and some severe cases have been treated with pulmonary vasodilators.[52]

GROUP 5.4: OTHER DISORDERS

Group 5.4 (other disorders) encompasses PH caused by chronic renal failure (CRF), fibrosing mediastinitis, tumor emboli, and mechanical vascular obstruction. Only PH associated with CRF is discussed.

Chronic Renal Failure on Dialysis

Incidence/etiology

The true incidence of PH CRF on dialysis is not known; however, prior studies relying on echocardiographically defined PH have reported that PH is common and associated with increased mortality. The etiology is multifactorial, including pulmonary venous hypertension secondary to left ventricular dysfunction, hypervolemia, and high-output secondary to anemia or shunting from an arteriovenous fistula.[53] CRF may also have a direct effect on the pulmonary vasculature due to systemic imbalances in vasoconstrictors and vasodilators, endothelial dysfunction, and vascular calcification.[53–55]

Treatment

The evaluation of PH in patients with CRF on dialysis depends on symptoms and clinical circumstances. Patients with more than mild PH (pulmonary arterial systolic pressure >50 mm Hg), with significant RV dysfunction on echocardiography, with systemic hypotension limiting fluid removal via hemodialysis, and who are considered for kidney transplantation should undergo RHC to understand etiology and guide treatment. Management consists of treating left ventricular systolic or diastolic dysfunction, optimizing fluid balance to achieve euvolemia, iron/erythropoietin supplementation to avoid anemia, and phosphate binders to limit vascular calcification. Clinical investigation of PAH therapies in CRF is needed.

SUMMARY

Group 5 PH consists of a complex group of disorders that are associated with PH. The cause is often multifactorial and can be secondary to increased precapillary and postcapillary pressure as well as direct effects on pulmonary vasculature. The true incidence of PH in these disorders is often unknown; however, studies suggest PH can be common and its presence is often associated with increased morbidity and mortality. Studies investigating the treatment of group 5 PH are rare and involve a limited number of patients; thus, management is guided by small case reports and series. In general, treatment is directed toward treating the underlying disorder. The etiology of PH should be thoroughly assessed in these patients, and treatment should be individually tailored to each patient. PAH therapies may have a role in some specific disease states on a case-by-case basis; however, patients must be carefully and fully assessed for the cause of their PH because the benefits of PAH therapies remain unclear and require further investigation.

REFERENCES

1. Simonneau G, Robbins IM, Beghetti M, et al. Updated clinical classification of pulmonary hypertension. J Am Coll Cardiol 2009;54(1 Suppl):S43–54.
2. Hoeper MM, Bogaard HJ, Condliffe R, et al. Definitions and diagnosis of pulmonary hypertension. J Am Coll Cardiol 2013;62(25 Suppl):D42–50.
3. Garypidou V, Vakalopoulou S, Dimitriadis D, et al. Incidence of pulmonary hypertension in patients with chronic myeloproliferative disorders. Haematologica 2004;89(2):245–6.
4. Galiè N, Humbert M, Vachiery JL, et al. 2015 ESC/ERS guidelines for the diagnosis and treatment of pulmonary hypertension: the Joint Task Force for the diagnosis and treatment of pulmonary hypertension of the European Society of Cardiology (ESC) and the European Respiratory Society (ERS) Endorsed by: Association for European Paediatric and Congenital Cardiology (AEPC), International Society for Heart and Lung Transplantation (ISHLT). Eur Heart J 2015;46(4):903–75.
5. Adir Y, Elia D, Harari S. Pulmonary hypertension in patients with chronic myeloproliferative disorders. Eur Respir Rev 2015;24(137):400–10.
6. Landolfi R, Di Gennaro L, Falanga A. Thrombosis in myeloproliferative disorders: pathogenetic facts and speculation. Leukemia 2008;22(11):2020–8.
7. Orlandi EM, Rocca B, Pazzano AS, et al. Reversible pulmonary arterial hypertension likely related to long-term, low-dose dasatinib treatment for chronic myeloid leukaemia. Leuk Res 2012;36(1):e4–6.
8. Cortelazzo S, Finazzi G, Ruggeri M, et al. Hydroxyurea for patients with essential thrombocythemia and a high risk of thrombosis. N Engl J Med 1995; 332(17):1132–6.

9. Tabarroki A, Lindner DJ, Visconte V, et al. Ruxolitinib leads to improvement of pulmonary hypertension in patients with myelofibrosis. Leukemia 2014;28(7):1486–93.

10. Low AT, Howard L, Harrison C, et al. Pulmonary arterial hypertension exacerbated by ruxolitinib. Haematologica 2015;100(6):e244–5.

11. Jaïs X, Ioos V, Jardim C, et al. Splenectomy and chronic thromboembolic pulmonary hypertension. Thorax 2005;60(12):1031–4.

12. Coltheart G, Little JM. Splenectomy: a review of morbidity. Aust N Z J Surg 1976;46(1):32–6.

13. Bonderman D, Wilkens H, Wakounig S, et al. Risk factors for chronic thromboembolic pulmonary hypertension. Eur Respir J 2009;33(2):325–31.

14. Mohren M, Markmann I, Dworschak U, et al. Thromboembolic complications after splenectomy for hematologic diseases. Am J Hematol 2004;76(2):143–7.

15. Atichartakarn V, Angchaisuksiri P, Aryurachai K, et al. Relationship between hypercoagulable state and erythrocyte phosphatidylserine exposure in splenectomized haemoglobin E/beta-thalassaemic patients. Br J Haematol 2002;118(3):893–8.

16. Piazza G, Goldhaber SZ. Chronic thromboembolic pulmonary hypertension. N Engl J Med 2011;364(4):351–60.

17. Jaïs X, D'Armini AM, Jansa P, et al. Bosentan for treatment of inoperable chronic thromboembolic pulmonary hypertension: BENEFiT (Bosentan Effects in iNopErable Forms of chronIc Thromboembolic pulmonary hypertension), a randomized, placebo-controlled trial. J Am Coll Cardiol 2008;52(25):2127–34.

18. Ghofrani HA, D'Armini AM, Grimminger F, et al. Riociguat for the treatment of chronic thromboembolic pulmonary hypertension. N Engl J Med 2013;369(4):319–29.

19. Bunn HF. Pathogenesis and treatment of sickle cell disease. N Engl J Med 1997;337(11):762–9.

20. Fonseca GH, Souza R, Salemi VM, et al. Pulmonary hypertension diagnosed by right heart catheterisation in sickle cell disease. Eur Respir J 2012;39(1):112–8.

21. Parent F, Bachir D, Inamo J, et al. A hemodynamic study of pulmonary hypertension in sickle cell disease. N Engl J Med 2011;365(1):44–53.

22. Mehari A, Gladwin MT, Tian X, et al. Mortality in adults with sickle cell disease and pulmonary hypertension. JAMA 2012;307(12):1254–6.

23. Reiter CD, Wang X, Tanus-Santos JE, et al. Cell-free hemoglobin limits nitric oxide bioavailability in sickle-cell disease. Nat Med 2002;8(12):1383–9.

24. Machado RF, Farber HW. Pulmonary hypertension associated with chronic hemolytic anemia and other blood disorders. Clin Chest Med 2013;34(4):739–52.

25. Anthi A, Machado RF, Jison ML, et al. Hemodynamic and functional assessment of patients with sickle cell disease and pulmonary hypertension. Am J Respir Crit Care Med 2007;175(12):1272–9.

26. Machado RF, Barst RJ, Yovetich NA, et al. Hospitalization for pain in patients with sickle cell disease treated with sildenafil for elevated TRV and low exercise capacity. Blood 2011;118(4):855–64.

27. Barst RJ, Mubarak KK, Machado RF, et al. Exercise capacity and haemodynamics in patients with sickle cell disease with pulmonary hypertension treated with bosentan: results of the ASSET studies. Br J Haematol 2010;149(3):426–35.

28. Castro O, Hoque M, Brown BD. Pulmonary hypertension in sickle cell disease: cardiac catheterization results and survival. Blood 2003;101(4):1257–61.

29. Aessopos A, Farmakis D. Pulmonary hypertension in beta-thalassemia. Ann N Y Acad Sci 2005;1054:342–9.

30. Atichartakarn V, Chuncharunee S, Chandanamattha P, et al. Correction of hypercoagulability and amelioration of pulmonary arterial hypertension by chronic blood transfusion in an asplenic hemoglobin E/beta-thalassemia patient. Blood 2004;103(7):2844–6.

31. Morris CR, Kim HY, Wood J, et al. Sildenafil therapy in thalassemia patients with Doppler-defined risk of pulmonary hypertension. Haematologica 2013;98(9):1359–67.

32. Anthi A, Tsangaris I, Hamodraka ES, et al. Treatment with bosentan in a patient with thalassemia intermedia and pulmonary arterial hypertension. Blood 2012;120(7):1531–2.

33. Handa T, Nagai S, Miki S, et al. Incidence of pulmonary hypertension and its clinical relevance in patients with sarcoidosis. Chest 2006;129(5):1246–52.

34. Shorr AF, Davies DB, Nathan SD. Predicting mortality in patients with sarcoidosis awaiting lung transplantation. Chest 2003;124(3):922–8.

35. Bourbonnais JM, Samavati L. Clinical predictors of pulmonary hypertension in sarcoidosis. Eur Respir J 2008;32(2):296–302.

36. Barst RJ, McGoon M, Torbicki A, et al. Diagnosis and differential assessment of pulmonary arterial hypertension. J Am Coll Cardiol 2004;43(12 Suppl S):40S–7S.

37. Corte TJ, Wells AU, Nicholson AG, et al. Pulmonary hypertension in sarcoidosis: a review. Respirology 2011;16(1):69–77.

38. Takemura T, Matsui Y, Saiki S, et al. Pulmonary vascular involvement in sarcoidosis: a report of 40 autopsy cases. Hum Pathol 1992;23(11):1216–23.

39. Nunes H, Freynet O, Naggara N, et al. Cardiac sarcoidosis. Semin Respir Crit Care Med 2010;31(4):428–41.

40. Preston IR, Klinger JR, Landzberg MJ, et al. Vasoresponsiveness of sarcoidosis-associated pulmonary hypertension. Chest 2001;120(3):866–72.

41. Milman N, Svendsen CB, Iversen M, et al. Sarcoidosis-associated pulmonary hypertension: acute

vasoresponsiveness to inhaled nitric oxide and the relation to long-term effect of sildenafil. Clin Respir J 2009;3(4):207–13.

42. Bonham CA, Oldham JM, Gomberg-Maitland M, et al. Therapy in sarcoidosis-associated pulmonary hypertension: a retrospective case series. Chest 2015;148(4):1055–62.

43. Le Pavec J, Lorillon G, Jaïs X, et al. Pulmonary Langerhans cell histiocytosis-associated pulmonary hypertension: clinical characteristics and impact of pulmonary arterial hypertension therapies. Chest 2012;142(5):1150–7.

44. Fartoukh M, Humbert M, Capron F, et al. Severe pulmonary hypertension in histiocytosis X. Am J Respir Crit Care Med 2000;161(1):216–23.

45. Li JH, Safford RE, Aduen JF, et al. Pulmonary hypertension and thyroid disease. Chest 2007;132(3): 793–7.

46. Chu JW, Kao PN, Faul JL, et al. High prevalence of autoimmune thyroid disease in pulmonary arterial hypertension. Chest 2002;122(5):1668–73.

47. Vallabhajosula S, Radhi S, Cevik C, et al. Hyperthyroidism and pulmonary hypertension: an important association. Am J Med Sci 2011;342(6):507–12.

48. Chadha C, Pritzker M, Mariash CN. Effect of epoprostenol on the thyroid gland: enlargement and secretion of thyroid hormone. Endocr Pract 2009; 15(2):116–21.

49. Marvisi M, Balzarini L, Mancini C, et al. Thyroid gland and pulmonary hypertension. What's the link? Panminerva Med 2013;55(1):93–7.

50. Humbert M, Labrune P, Simonneau G. Severe pulmonary arterial hypertension in type 1 glycogen storage disease. Eur J Pediatr 2002;161(Suppl 1):S93–6.

51. Smith RL, Hutchins GM, Sack GH, et al. Unusual cardiac, renal and pulmonary involvement in Gaucher's disease. Intersitial glucocerebroside accumulation, pulmonary hypertension and fatal bone marrow embolization. Am J Med 1978;65(2):352–60.

52. Mistry PK, Sirrs S, Chan A, et al. Pulmonary hypertension in type 1 Gaucher's disease: genetic and epigenetic determinants of phenotype and response to therapy. Mol Genet Metab 2002;77(1–2):91–8.

53. Sise ME, Courtwright AM, Channick RN. Pulmonary hypertension in patients with chronic and end-stage kidney disease. Kidney Int 2013;84(4):682–92.

54. Abdelwhab S, Elshinnawy S. Pulmonary hypertension in chronic renal failure patients. Am J Nephrol 2008;28(6):990–7.

55. Dhaun N, Goddard J, Webb DJ. The endothelin system and its antagonism in chronic kidney disease. J Am Soc Nephrol 2006;17(4):943–55.

Pulmonary Hypertension in Children

Dunbar Ivy, MD

KEYWORDS

• Pulmonary arterial hypertension • Single-ventricle circulation • Bronchopulmonary dysplasia

KEY POINTS

- The prevalence of PH is increasing in the pediatric population, because of improved recognition and increased survival of patients, and remains a significant cause of morbidity and mortality.
- Recent studies have improved the understanding of pediatric PH, but management remains challenging because of a lack of evidence-based clinical trials.
- The growing recognition of developmental lung disease associated with PH requires dedicated research to explore the use of existing therapies as well as the creation of novel therapies.
- Adequate study of pediatric PH will require multicenter collaboration due to the small numbers of patients, multifactorial disease causes, and practice variability.

INTRODUCTION

Untreated, pulmonary arterial hypertension (PAH) in children carries a particularly poor prognosis. In the National Institutes of Health registry, the median untreated survival for children after diagnosis of idiopathic PAH (IPAH) was reported to be 10 months as opposed to 2.8 years for adults.[1] In 1999, further studies by Barst and colleagues[2] showed that survival for children with IPAH who were candidates for intravenous prostacyclin but were unable to be treated with this therapy was poor with a survival of 45% and 29%, respectively, at 1 and 4 years. Recent advances in the understanding of the pathobiology of IPAH and new treatment therapies have resulted in marked improvement in the prognosis for children with PAH (**Fig. 1**).[3,4] Similarities and differences persist in comparison of children and adults with PAH.[5] In both groups, disease progression is rapid, perhaps more rapid in children than in adults, and left untreated, elevation of pulmonary arterial pressure (PAP) and resistance leads to right ventricular (RV) failure, clinical deterioration, and death. In contrast, many aspects of pulmonary vascular disease of children are distinct from adult

pulmonary hypertension (PH). Pediatric PH is intrinsically linked to lung growth and development in the younger child as defined in the Panama classification (**Box 1**, **Fig. 2**).[6] The onset of pulmonary vascular injury in the younger child may allow the possibility of greater reversal of pulmonary vascular disease, particularly in bronchopulmonary dysplasia (BPD) and other lung diseases of childhood. Medical management of children follows a similar algorithm to that of adults treated with idiopathic pulmonary vascular disease.[4,7,8] The resurgence of the Potts shunt, originally used to increase pulmonary blood flow in congenital heart disease (CHD) in the 1950s, has allowed for a surgical right-to-left shunt in the younger child failing medical management with end-stage disease.[9]

DEFINITION

Similar to adults, PAH is defined as a mean PAP greater than 25 mm Hg at rest, with a normal pulmonary artery wedge pressure less than 15 mm Hg and an increased pulmonary vascular resistance (PVR) greater than 3 Wood units × M[2].[4,10] Both the Nice and Panama classifications are

Section of Pediatric Cardiology, Children's Hospital Colorado, University of Colorado School of Medicine, 13123 East 16th Avenue, B100, Aurora, CO 80045, USA
E-mail address: dunbar.ivy@childrenscolorado.org

Cardiol Clin 34 (2016) 451–472
http://dx.doi.org/10.1016/j.ccl.2016.04.005
0733-8651/16/$ – see front matter © 2016 Elsevier Inc. All rights reserved.

cardiology.theclinics.com

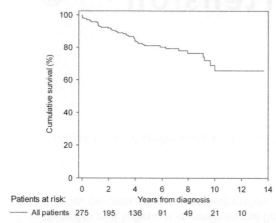

Fig. 1. Kaplan-Meier curves showing the survival pediatric PAH patients at 3 PH centers (NY, New York; NL, Netherlands): 1-, 3-, 5-, and 7-year transplantation-free survival rates were 96%, 89%, 81%, and 79%, respectively. (*From* Zijlstra WM, Douwes JM, Rosenzweig EB. Survival differences in pediatric pulmonary arterial hypertension: clues to a better understanding of outcome and optimal treatment strategies. J Am Coll Cardiol 2014;63(20):2159–69; with permission.)

appropriate for adults and children.[4,11] In younger children, the PAP is frequently referenced as a ratio to systemic arterial pressure with a significant difference being greater than 0.5. Pulmonary

hypertensive vascular disease complicates the course of certain forms of single-ventricle heart disease in which mean PAP is less than 25 mm Hg, but PVR is high, leading to failure of the circulation.[6] PAH associated with CHD is heterogeneous and ranges from classic Eisenmenger syndrome with reversal of a central shunt and cyanosis to IPAH-like CHD with coincidental defects (**Box 2**).[11]

EPIDEMIOLOGY

National registries from the United Kingdom, the Netherlands, and Spain have all shown a lower incidence for IPAH in children compared with adults. The incidence of IPAH in the national registry from the United Kingdom was 0.48 cases per million children per year, and the prevalence was 2.1 cases per million.[12] In the Netherlands, annual incidence and point prevalence averaged 0.7 and 2.2 cases per million children, respectively (**Fig. 3**).[13] Likewise, in the Spanish registry, the incidence and prevalence were 0.49 and 2.9 cases per million children.[14] PAH associated with CHD represents highly heterogeneous subgroups. Transient PAH is seen in children with CHD and systemic-to-pulmonary shunt, in whom PAH resolves after early shunt correction. However, in a small subset of CHD progressive PAH after surgical repair associated PAH (APAH)-CHD Group D (**Box 2**) has a particularly poor diagnosis (**Fig. 4**).[15] APAH-CHD occurs more frequently in children than adults with an incidence and

---

Box 1
Developmental lung diseases associated with pulmonary hypertension

- Congenital diaphragmatic hernia
- Bronchopulmonary dysplasia
- Alveolar capillary dysplasia (ACD)
- ACD with misalignment of veins
- Lung hypoplasia ("primary" or "secondary")
- Surfactant protein abnormalities
  - ○ Surfactant protein B deficiency
  - ○ Surfactant protein C deficiency
  - ○ ATP-binding cassette A3 mutation
  - ○ Thyroid transcription factor 1/Nkx2.1 homeobox mutation
- Pulmonary interstitial glycogenosis
- Pulmonary alveolar proteinosis
- Pulmonary lymphangiectasia

From Ivy DD, Abman SH, Barst RJ, et al. Pediatric pulmonary hypertension. J Am Coll Cardiol 2013;62(Suppl 25):D117–26; with permission.

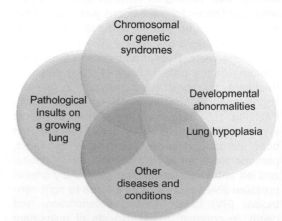

Fig. 2. Venn diagram illustrating the heterogeneity and multifactorial elements in pediatric pulmonary hypertensive vascular disease. (*Adapted from* Cerro MJ, Abman S, Diaz G, et al. A consensus approach to the classification of pediatric pulmonary hypertensive vascular disease: report from the PVRI Pediatric Taskforce, Panama 2011. Pulm Circ 2011;1(2):286–98; with permission.)

Box 2
Updated clinical classification of pulmonary arterial hypertension associated with congenital heart disease

A. Eisenmenger syndrome

Includes all large intracardiac and extracardiac defects, which begin as systemic-to-pulmonary shunts and progress with time to severe elevation of PVR and to reversal (pulmonary-to-systemic) or bidirectional shunting; cyanosis, secondary erythrocytosis, and multiple organ involvement are usually present.

B. Left-to-right shunts

- Correctable
- Noncorrectable

Include moderate-to-large defects; PVR is mildly to moderately increased; systemic-to-pulmonary shunting is still prevalent, whereas cyanosis is not a feature.

C. PAH with coincidental congenital heart disease

Marked elevation in PVR in the presence of small cardiac defects, which themselves do not account for the development of elevated PVR; the clinical picture is very similar to IPAH. Closing the defects is contraindicated.

D. Postoperative PAH

Congenital heart disease is repaired but PAH either persists immediately after surgery or recurs/develops months or years after surgery in the absence of significant postoperative hemodynamic lesions. The clinical phenotype is often aggressive.

From Simonneau G, Gatzoulis MA, Adatia I, et al. Updated clinical classification of pulmonary hypertension. J Am Coll Cardiol 2013;62(Suppl 25):D34–41; with permission.

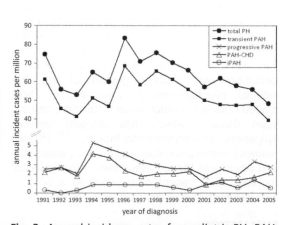

Fig. 3. Annual incidence rates for pediatric PH. PAH-CHD, PAH associated with congenital heart defects. (*From* van Loon RL, Roofthooft MT, Hillege HL, et al. Pediatric pulmonary hypertension in the Netherlands: epidemiology and characterization during the period 1991 to 2005. Circulation 2011;124(16):1755–64; with permission.)

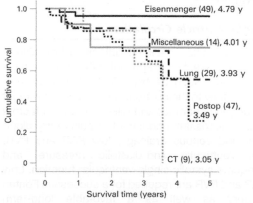

Fig. 4. Survival curves for the subgroups within the associated pulmonary arterial hypertension (APAH) group from the UK PH service. The number in each group (*parentheses*) and the predicted survival out of a possible 5 years is depicted. Note, the worst survival for children is with postoperative CHD. CT, computed tomography. (*From* Haworth SG, Hislop AA. Treatment and survival in children with pulmonary arterial hypertension: the UK Pulmonary Hypertension Service for children 2001-2006. Heart 2009;95(4):312–7; with permission.)

prevalence 2.2 and 15.6 cases per million children. Syndromes are frequently present in progressive PAH. Recent national database studies have suggested an increasing prevalence of hospitalized children with PH as a comorbidity. Increased recognition of pediatric PH may also play a role.[16,17]

HIGHLIGHTED CAUSES OF PULMONARY HYPERTENSION
Heritable Pulmonary Arterial Hypertension

Bone morphogenetic protein receptor type 2 (*BMPR2*) mutations have been identified in children and adults with IPAH and familial PAH.[18–24] The pattern of inheritance in children with *BMPR2* mutations is the same as adults with an autosomal-dominant pattern with reduced penetrance. *BMPR2* mutations have been evaluated in several pediatric series with inconsistent results. Grunig and colleagues[24] found no BMPR2 mutations or deletions in 13 children with IPAH. However, in a study by Harrison and colleagues,[21] 22% of children with IPAH or PH associated with CHD had activin-like kinase type-1 (*ALK-1*) or *BMPR2* mutations. In a Japanese study, children with severe heritable pulmonary arterial hypertension (HPAH) were as likely to have a BMPR2 mutation as an ALK-1 mutation.[25] Advanced gene-sequencing methods have facilitated the discovery of additional genes with mutations among those with and those without familial forms of PAH (*SMAD-9*, *CAV1*, *KCNK3*, *EIF2AK4*, *TBX4*).[18,26–28]

Single-Ventricle Circulation

PVR plays a key role in the outcome of the single-ventricle patient. In the patient with single-ventricle physiology, such as hypoplastic left heart syndrome, flow to the pulmonary circulation is without a pumping chamber and relies on several factors to be successful: unobstructed pulmonary blood flow and venous drainage, low PAP and PVR, low ventricular end-diastolic pressure, and adequate systolic single-ventricular function. Low PAP and PVR are required for a successful Fontan surgery as well as a favorable long-term outcome.[29] Increases in PAP and PVR lead to abnormalities of the systemic and pulmonary circulations. High PVR leads to low cardiac output and is associated with Fontan failure as well as complications such as protein-losing enteropathy[30] and plastic bronchitis.[31] Risk factors for palliation failure include mean PAP greater than 15 mm Hg, transpulmonary gradient greater than 8 mm Hg, and indexed pulmonary vascular resistance (PVRI) greater than 2.5 Wood U $\times$ m^2.[32] Pulmonary

vascular disease with muscular thickening of the pulmonary arteries and an overexpression of nitric oxide (NO) synthase has been found in patients with a failing Fontan circulation.[33] Likewise, children receiving a heart transplant for Fontan failure have an elevated PVR 1 year after transplantation.[34]

Based on the above observations, treatment of the Fontan patient with pulmonary vasodilator therapy in small series has been shown to improve hemodynamics and saturation, exercise capacity, and treat complications, such as protein-losing enteropathy and plastic bronchitis in the "failing" and "nonfailing" Fontan patient.[35–37] The vasoconstrictor peptide endothelin-1 (ET-1) is increased in Fontan patients.[38] Several studies have suggested an exercise benefit with ET receptor antagonists.[39–41]

Bronchopulmonary Dysplasia

BPD is the chronic lung disease associated with prematurity and is one of the many developmental lung diseases of childhood associated with PH (**Box 3, Fig. 5**). Advances in neonatal care have improved survival of extremely premature infants, but morbidity from BPD is significant, and PH is diagnosed in up to 20% of preterm babies.[42] PH is associated with mild, moderate, and severe BPD, with increasing PH associated with worse BPD (**Fig. 5**). PH is usually diagnosed by echocardiogram, but the variable rates of PH diagnosis are likely related to lack of consistent echocardiographic criteria. However, early echocardiographic signs of pulmonary vascular disease as early as 7 days of life (ventricular septal wall flattening and right ventricle dilation) are associated with higher risk of late PH in preterm infants at risk of BPD.[43] PH is thought to result from increased vascular tone, hypertensive remodeling, and a limited vascular bed. Risk factors for PH include lower gestational age, small-for-gestational age birth weight, oligohydramnios, preeclampsia, prolonged duration of mechanical ventilation, and oxygen therapy, which may suggest genetic, epigenetic, or environmental factors.[42–45] PH can resolve in some premature infants, and persistence and severity of PH are associated with significant mortality. One recent study showed a 53% $\pm$ 11% survival 2 years after diagnosis of PH.[46]

EVALUATION

Recent guidelines on the diagnosis and management of children with PH have filled gaps in evaluation and treatment of children with PH.[44] A complete evaluation for all possible causes of PAH is required before the diagnosis of IPAH is

Box 3
Select guidelines from the American Heart Association and American Thoracic Society Task Force

Diagnosis, assessments, monitoring

1. After a comprehensive initial evaluation, serial echocardiograms should be performed. More frequent echocardiograms are recommended in the setting of changes in therapy or clinical condition (class I; level of evidence B).

2. Cardiac catheterization is recommended before initiation of PAH-targeted therapy (class I; level of evidence B). Exceptions may include critically ill patients requiring immediate initiation of empirical therapy (class I; level of evidence B).

3. Cardiac catheterization should include acute vasoreactivity testing (AVT) unless there is a specific contraindication (class I; level of evidence A).

4. Repeat cardiac catheterization is recommended within 3 to 12 months after initiation of therapy to evaluate response or with clinical worsening (class I; level of evidence B).

5. BNP or NT proBNP should be measured at diagnosis and during follow-up to supplement clinical decision (class I; level of evidence B).

6. Recommendations for genetic testing of first-degree relatives of patients with monogenic forms of HPAH include the following:

   a. Genetic testing is indicated for risk stratification (class I; level of evidence B).

   b. Members of families afflicted with HPAH who develop new cardiorespiratory symptoms should be evaluated immediately for PAH (class I; level of evidence B).

Bronchopulmonary dysplasia

1. Screening for PH by echocardiogram is recommended in infants with established BPD (class I; level of evidence B).

2. Evaluation and treatment of lung disease, including assessments for hypoxemia, aspiration, structural airway disease, and the need for changes in respiratory support, are recommended in infants with BPD and PH before initiation of PAH-targeted therapy (class I; level of evidence B).

3. Evaluation for long-term therapy for PH in infants with BPD should follow recommendations for all children with PH and include cardiac catheterization to diagnose disease severity and potential contributing factors such as LV diastolic dysfunction, anatomic shunts, pulmonary vein stenosis, and systemic collaterals (class I; level of evidence B).

4. PAH-targeted therapy can be useful for infants with BPD and PH on optimal treatment of underlying respiratory and cardiac disease (class IIa; level of evidence C).

Pharmacotherapy

1. Recommendations for CCBs include the following:

   a. CCBs should be given only to those patients who are reactive as assessed by AVT and greater than 1 year of age (class I; level of evidence C).

   b. CCBs are contraindicated in children who have not undergone or are nonresponsive to AVT and in patients with right-sided heart dysfunction owing to the potential for negative inotropic effects of CCB therapy (class III; level of evidence C).

2. Oral PAH-targeted therapy in children with lower-risk PAH is recommended and should include either a phosphodiesterase type 5 inhibitor or an ET receptor antagonist (class I; level of evidence B).

3. Intravenous and subcutaneous prostacyclin or its analogues should be initiated without delay for patients with higher-risk PAH (class I; level of evidence B).

4. Referral to lung transplantation centers for evaluation is recommended for patients who are in WHO-FC III or IV on optimized medical therapy or who have rapidly progressive disease (class I; level of evidence A).

Outpatient care of the child with pulmonary hypertension

1. The following preventive care measures for health maintenance are recommended for pediatric patients with PH (class I; level of evidence C):

   a. Respiratory syncytial virus prophylaxis (if eligible)

   b. Influenza and pneumococcal vaccinations

    c. Rigorous monitoring of growth parameters

    d. Prompt recognition and treatment of infectious respiratory illnesses

    e. Antibiotic prophylaxis for the prevention of subacute bacterial endocarditis in cyanotic patients and those with indwelling central lines

2. Because of the risks of syncope or sudden death with exertion, it is recommended that a thorough evaluation, including cardiopulmonary exercise testing and treatment, be performed before the patient engages in athletic (symptom-limited) activities (class I; level of evidence C).

3. Pediatric patients with severe PH (WHO-FC III or IV) or recent history of syncope should not participate in competitive sports (class III; level of evidence C).

4. During exercise, it is recommended that pediatric patients with PH engage in light to moderate aerobic activity, avoid strenuous and isometric exertion, remain well hydrated, and be allowed to self-limit as required (class I; level of evidence C).

From Abman SH, Hansmann G, Archer SL, et al. Pediatric pulmonary hypertension: guidelines from the American Heart Association and American Thoracic Society. Circulation 2015;132(21):2037–99. Reprinted with permission. © 2015 American Heart Association, Inc.

made (**Box 3**). Certain diseases, such as connective tissue disease or chronic thromboembolic PH, are less likely to be discovered in children, but still should be excluded. As discussed later, cardiac catheterization is required to rule out subtle CHD, such as pulmonary vein disease, to determine right atrial pressure, PAP, PVR, and vasoreactivity to acute vasodilator testing.[47] Lung biopsy is rarely performed but may be helpful to exclude certain diseases, such as pulmonary veno-occlusive disease, pulmonary capillary hemangiomatosis, or alveolar capillary dysplasia. Furthermore, in certain forms of interstitial lung disease, such as pulmonary capillaritis or hypersensitivity pneumonitis, lung biopsy may be beneficial because treatment of these disorders varies markedly from the approach used in IPAH.

Echocardiography is a very useful noninvasive screening tool to evaluate patients with a clinical suspicion of PAH.[48] The echocardiogram documents cardiac anatomy, RV size and function, left ventricular (LV) systolic and diastolic function, morphology and function of valves, and the presence of pericardial effusion or a patent foramen ovale. Doppler ultrasound can be used noninvasively to estimate the pulmonary artery systolic pressure and to suggest the presence of increased PVR. A qualitative assessment of RV function is also important; this is often challenging due to the geometry of the RV. Several measures are available to attempt to quantify the degree of RV dysfunction, including the Tei index (myocardial performance index), RV ejection fraction, RV fractional area change, and the tricuspid annular plane systolic excursion (TAPSE).[49–56] Normal values for TAPSE in children have recently been published and should serve as a reference for children with PH (**Fig. 6**).[52] The ratio of right ventricle to left ventricle size at end systole is a strong predictor of outcome (**Fig. 7**).[57] An increasing RV/LV systolic ratio (RV/LV) is associated with an increasing hazard for a clinical event (hazard ratio, 2.49; 95% confidence interval, 1.92–3.24). Pulmonic valve insufficiency is frequently seen, and characteristics of the pulmonic regurgitant flow velocity or changes in the systolic flow velocity profile across the pulmonic valve also can be used to estimate noninvasively the pulmonary artery diastolic pressure and the mean pulmonary artery pressure.[58] The presence of a pericardial effusion is rare in children, but when present, suggests a poor prognosis.[53,59] As PH progresses and RV function worsens, the systolic portion of the cardiac cycle lengthens, leading to an increase in the systolic:diastolic (S/D) ratio.

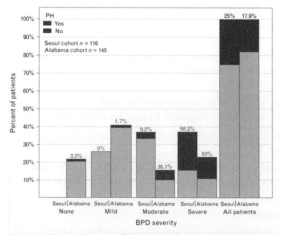

Fig. 5. The incidence of PH according to the degree of BPD severity. Numbers above the bars indicate the percentage of patients with PH. (*Data from* Refs.[172–174])

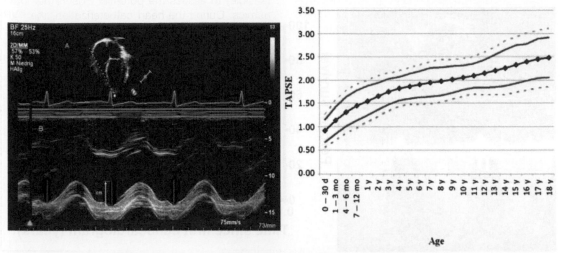

Fig. 6. Measurement and normal values for TAPSE. (*From* Koestenberger M, Ravekes W, Everett AD. Right ventricular function in infants, children and adolescents: reference values of the tricuspid annular plane systolic excursion (TAPSE) in 640 healthy patients and calculation of z score values. J Am Soc Echocardiogr 2009;22(6):715–9; with permission.)

The S/D ratio is higher in PH patients than in controls (1.38 ± 0.61 vs 0.72 ± 0.16, *P*<.001) and is associated with worse echocardiographic RV fractional area change, worse catheterization hemodynamics, shorter 6-minute walk (6MW) distance, and worse clinical outcomes independent of pulmonary resistance or pressures (**Fig. 8**).[56,60,61] Tissue Doppler imaging directly measures myocardial velocities and has been shown to be an accurate measure of RV and LV systolic and diastolic function. In recent pediatric studies, RV tissue Doppler imaging velocity was lower in children with PAH compared with healthy controls.[62,63] Moreover, tricuspid diastolic

velocity (E′) had significant inverse correlations with RV end-diastolic pressure and mean PAP, and cumulative event-free survival rate was significantly lower when tricuspid E′ velocity was 8 cm/s or less (log-rank test, *P*<.001; **Fig. 9**).[63] The right ventricle contracts primarily in a longitudinal fashion; thus RV longitudinal strain measurement may play an important role in evaluation of RV function. RV longitudinal strain is a powerful tool to predict clinical outcome in adults with PH.[64] Finally, real-time 3-dimensional echocardiography correlates well with cardiac MRI in children with CHD[65] and is being evaluated in children with PH.

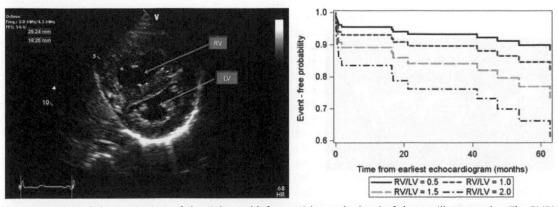

Fig. 7. Parasternal short-axis view of the right and left ventricles at the level of the papillary muscles. The RV/LV ratio is derived from RV diameter and LV diameter at end systole. RV/LV end-systole ratio is predictive of outcome. Estimated survival curves for 4 possible RV/LV ratios estimated from the Cox varying coefficients regression corresponding to a hazard ratio of 2.49 for RV/LV ratio. (*From* Jone PN, Hinzman J, Wagner BD, et al. Right ventricular to left ventricular diameter ratio at end-systole in evaluating outcomes in children with pulmonary hypertension. J Am Soc Echocardiogr 2014;27(2):172–8; with permission.)

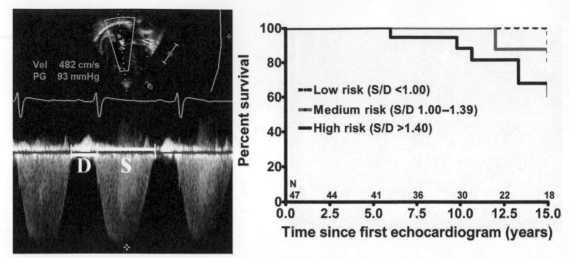

Fig. 8. The systolic (S) to diastolic (D) time ratio from tricuspid regurgitation velocity can be calculated as a measure of RV function. An increase in the S/D ratio predicts worse outcome in children with PH. Alkon and colleagues[60] in 2010 used a simple measure of S/D time ratio from the TR jet to evaluate pediatric PH patients and found that as the RV function worsens, the systolic portion of the cardiac cycle lengthens, leading to an increased S/D ratio. S/D ratio was found to be higher in PH patients compared with controls and is associated with worse RV fractional area change, worse hemodynamics by catheterization, shorter 6-minute walk test, and worse clinical outcomes independent of PVR or pressures. S/D ratio less than 1 was associated with low risk of poor outcome and S/D ratio greater than 1.4 was associated with high risk of negative outcome. Vel, velocity. (*From* Alkon J, Humpl T, Manlhiot C, et al. Usefulness of the right ventricular systolic to diastolic duration ration to predict functional capacity and survival in children with pulmonary arterial hypertension. Am J Cardiol 2010;106(3):430–6; with permission.)

Several additional tests may help quantitate exercise capacity and response to therapy. As in adults, the 6MW test is feasible and has been used to measure submaximal exercise. Unfortunately, the 6MW test has not been validated in children with PAH. In general, children with PAH tend to walk further than their adult counterparts with the same World Health Organization (WHO) functional class (FC), which may be partially explained by the less frequent prevalence of right heart failure in children. Normal values for 6MWD for children have recently been published.[66–69]

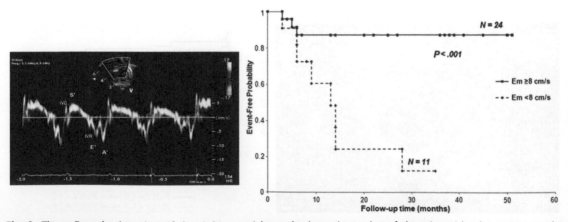

Fig. 9. Tissue Doppler imaging of the right ventricle at the lateral annulus of the tricuspid valve measures the myocardial systolic wave (S'), which measures the systolic longitudinal function of the RV and 2 diastolic waves: early diastolic (E') and late diastolic (A'), which denote the diastolic function of the ventricles. Low E' velocity less than 8 cm/s is predictive of poor outcome in pediatric IPAH. IVC, inferior vena cava. (*From* Takatsuki S, Nakayama T, Jone PN, et al. Tissue Doppler imaging predicts adverse outcome in children with idiopathic pulmonary arterial hypertension. J Pediatr 2012;161(6):1126–31; with permission.)

However, baseline 6MWD is not a predictor of survival, neither when expressed as an absolute distance in meters nor when adjusted to reference values expressed as z score or as percentage of predicted value.[12,70]

Cardiopulmonary exercise testing in children older than 7 years of age is useful to determine peak oxygen consumption, ventilator efficiency (VE) slope (Ve/VCO2), and anaerobic threshold.[71,72] VE slope is significantly higher in patients with PAH, with an estimated increase of 7.2 for each increase in WHO class, and correlates strongly with invasive measures of disease severity, including PAP, PVRI, and outcome.[73]

In adults, brain natriuretic peptide (BNP) is a useful tool to assess mortality risk, progression of the disease, and response to therapy.[74] Recent studies in children have begun to identify usefulness of BNP or N-terminal pro-brain natriuretic peptide (NT-proBNP).[75–77] Furthermore, change in BNP measurements over time correlates with the change in the hemodynamic and echocardiographic parameters of children with PAH; with a BNP value greater than 180 pg/mL predicting a decreased survival rate (**Fig. 10**). The change in BNP level in a specific patient over time was shown to be more helpful in determining risk or hemodynamic response to therapy than the average value in a pediatric PAH population.[76]

Although biomarkers may be used as treatment goals, to be useful, treatment-induced improvements in these variables should be associated with improved survival. In the Netherlands national registry, WHO-FC, NT-proBNP, and TAPSE were identified as follow-up predictors in which treatment-induced changes were associated with survival. Patients in whom these variables improved after treatment showed better survival.[78]

Newer techniques have begun to evaluate RV function by determination of total RV afterload by measuring impedance, cardiac MRI, and 3-dimensional echocardiography. PVR is the current standard for evaluating reactivity in children with PAH. However, PVR measures only the mean component of RV afterload and neglects pulsatile effects. Total RV afterload can be measured as pulmonary vascular input impedance and consists of a dynamic component (compliance/stiffness) and a static component (resistance).[79–81] In children, pulsatile components of RV afterload, represented by pulmonary arterial capacitance and pulmonary stroke volume index, provide important prognostic information to conventional static hemodynamic parameters.[82,83] RV stroke work (RVSW), the product of mean pulmonary artery pressure and stroke volume, integrates contractility, afterload, and ventricular-vascular coupling. RVSW can be estimated in children with PAH by echocardiography or catheterization and is significantly associated with abnormal WHO-FC, the need for atrial septostomy, as well as mortality.[84,85] Evaluation of MRI parameters in children with PAH has shown that RV ejection fraction and LV stroke volume index were most strongly predictive of survival on

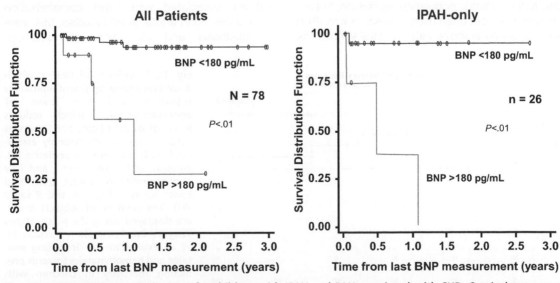

Fig. 10. Kaplan-Meier survival curves for children with IPAH and PAH associated with CHD. Survival curves are shown for all patients (*left*) and for the subgroup of IPAH patients (*right*) categorized with either BNP >180 pg/mL or less than 180 pg/mL. (*From* Bernus A, Wagner BD, Accurso F, et al. Brain natriuretic peptide levels in managing pediatric patients with pulmonary arterial hypertension. Chest 2009;135(3):745–51; with permission.)

univariate analysis (2.6- and 2.5-fold increase in mortality for every 1 SD decrease, respectively).[86]

Inflammation is an important contributor to PAH in children as it is in adults.[87,88] Serum amyloid A-4 (an acute phase protein released in response to inflammatory stimuli) was 4-fold higher in children with poor outcome (death, initiation of intravenous prostacyclin) compared with those with good outcome (survival, discontinuation of intravenous prostacyclin).[89] Interleukin-6, a proinflammatory cytokine, is associated with the occurrence of an adverse event in pediatric PH.[90] Inflammatory cells, such as fibrocytes and myeloid-derived suppressor cells (MDSCs), are increased in inflammatory disease and orchestrate immune cell responses. Recent published studies have shown that circulating fibrocytes and MDSCs were increased in 26 children with PAH compared with non-PAH controls.[91] High levels of tissue inhibitors of metalloproteinases-1 (TIMP-1), which is overexpressed by proinflammatory cytokines, and low levels of apolipoprotein-A1,[92] which reduces levels of oxidized lipids and improves vascular disease, are strongly associated with outcome in pediatric PH (Fig. 11).[93]

CONVENTIONAL THERAPY

Conventional therapy in patients used to treat RV failure is frequently used in PAH in children. Digoxin is used in the presence of RV failure, although there are no clear-cut data in children. Furthermore, warfarin and other antithrombotic agents are used to prevent thrombosis in situ, although data specific to the pediatric population are lacking. Anticoagulation is more often used in children with IPAH and especially in those with a central venous line for intravenous prostanoid therapy or those with a hypercoagulable state. In adults and children with IPAH who receive anticoagulation, low-dose warfarin is frequently used to target an INR of 1.5 to 2.[94] Diuretics are used to treat peripheral edema or ascites in the presence of right heart failure, but excessive diuresis should be avoided. Careful attention to respiratory tract infections is required because this may worsen alveolar hypoxia. Routine influenza vaccination as well as pneumococcal vaccination is recommended. The use of decongestants with pseudoephedrine or other stimulant-type medications should be avoided because these have been associated with PAH.[95] In children who require the use of oral contraceptive agents either for prevention of pregnancy or for regulation of menses, agents that have no estrogen content should be used. Pulse oximetry and polysomnography are indicated, and chronic hypoxemia or nighttime desaturation is aggressively treated. However, oxygen therapy is not used as a mainstay of therapy in children with normal daytime saturations. In the presence of resting hypoxemia, chronic supplemental oxygen may be used.

VASOREACTIVITY TESTING

Cardiac catheterization with acute vasodilator testing is essential before selecting targeted therapy in children. Cardiac catheterization carries a greater risk in those children with baseline suprasystemic PAP (odds ratio = 8.1, P = .02).[96,97] In the TOPP (Tracking Outcomes and Practice in Pediatric Pulmonary Hypertension) registry, complications associated with heart catheterization were analyzed in a total of 908 studies: 554 were at diagnosis and 354 were at follow-up.

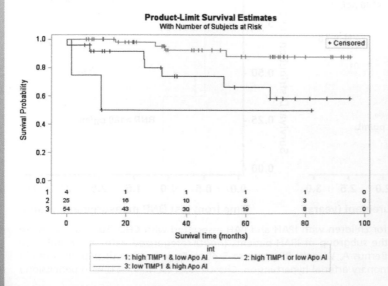

Product-Limit Survival Estimates
With Number of Subjects at Risk

Fig. 11. High levels of TIMP-1, which is overexpressed by proinflammatory cytokines, and low levels of apolipoprotein-A1, which reduces levels of oxidied lipids and improves vascular disease are strongly associated with outcome in pediatric PH. Patients with high TIMP-1 and low apolipoprotein-AI values (red) had lower survival (log-rank test P value .01). The number of subjects at-risk are displayed along the x-axis. (From Wagner BD, Takatsuki S, Accurso FJ, et al. Evaluation of circulating proteins and hemodynamics towards predicting mortality in children with pulmonary arterial hypertension. PLoS One 2013;8(11):e80235; with permission.)

Complications were reported in 5.9% with 5 deaths considered related to catheterization, suggesting a higher rate of catheterization complications compared with adult studies.[47] As in adults, a short-acting vasodilator is used, such as inhaled NO.[2,98,99] It is unclear at this time whether the criteria for acute vasoreactivity are the same in adults as in children.[2,3,100,101] There was no difference in the number of vasoreactivity responders in children with IPAH using the Barst or Sitbon criteria in a Netherlands study (**Fig. 12**).[100]

PHARMACOLOGIC THERAPY OF PULMONARY ARTERIAL HYPERTENSION

Based on known mechanisms of action, 3 classes of drugs have been extensively studied for the treatment of IPAH in adults: prostanoids, which stimulate cyclic adenosine monophosphate (epoprostenol, treprostinil, iloprost, beraprost); ET receptor antagonists, which block ET (bosentan, ambrisentan, macitentan); and drugs that stimulate the NO-cyclic guanosine monophosphate (cGMP) system (phosphodiesterase inhibitors: sildenafil, tadalafil; soluble guanylate cyclase [sGC] stimulators: riociguat). A pediatric-specific treatment algorithm, which applies mostly to children

with IPAH, was developed at the World Symposium of Pulmonary Hypertension in Nice 2013, and a recent adaptation is presented incorporating newer pharmaceutical therapies and surgical approaches (**Fig. 13, Table 1**).[4]

CALCIUM CHANNEL BLOCKERS

The use of calcium channel antagonists to evaluate vasoreactivity is dangerous, because these drugs can cause a decrease in cardiac output or a marked drop in systemic blood pressure. Such deleterious effects may be prolonged because of the relatively long half-life of calcium channel blockers. Consequently, elevated right atrial pressure and low cardiac output are contraindications to acute or chronic calcium channel blockade. Recent data have shown that 10% to 35% of children with IPAH are responders to acute vasodilator testing.[4,15,100,102]

An acute trial of calcium channel blocker therapy should only be used in those patients who are acutely responsive to either NO or prostacyclin. Likewise, patients who do not have an acute vasodilatory response to short-acting agents and who are then placed on calcium channel blocker therapy are unlikely to benefit from this form of

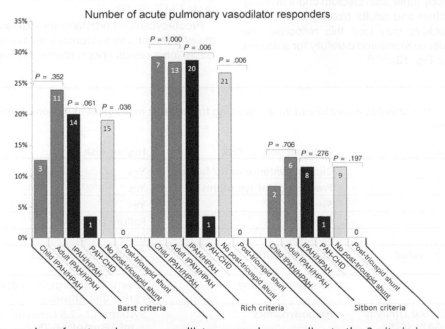

Fig. 12. The number of acute pulmonary vasodilator responders according to the 3 criteria in use, in children versus adults with IPAH/HPAH, IPAH/HPAH versus PAH associated with CHD, and patients without versus with posttricuspid shunt, respectively. Data presented as percentage of patient group (%) and patient numbers (indicated in bars). Comparison between groups performed using Fisher's exact test. Note the few percent of patients with PAH-CHD responding to acute vasodilator challenge. (*From* Douwes JM, van Loon RL, Hoendermis ES, et al. Acute pulmonary vasodilator response in paediatric and adult pulmonary arterial hypertension: occurrence and prognostic value when comparing three response criteria. Eur Heart J 2011;32(24):3137–46; with permission.)

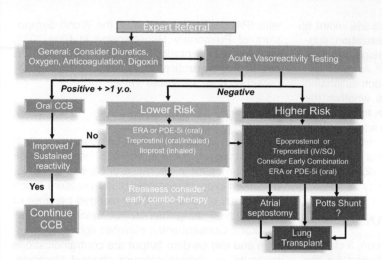

Fig. 13. Treatment algorithm proposed in the management of pediatric patients with idiopathic or heritable PAH. This may be translatable to other patients with PH. ERA, endothelin receptor antagonist; IV, intravenous; PDE-5i, phosphodiesterase 5 inhibitor; SQ, subcutaneous. Use of all agents is considered off label in children aside from sildenafil in the European Union. (*Data from* Ivy DD, Abman SH, Barst RJ, et al. Pediatric pulmonary hypertension. J Am Coll Cardiol 2013;62(Suppl 25):D117–26; with permission.)

therapy.[2] Recent study examined a previously identified cohort of 77 children diagnosed between 1982 and 1995 with IPAH and followed up through 2002. For acute responders treated with calcium channel blocker (CCB) (n = 31), survival at 1, 5, and 10 years was 97%, 97%, and 81%, respectively; treatment success was 84%, 68%, and 47%, respectively (see **Fig. 10**).[103] Sixty percent to 80% of children with severe PH are nonresponsive to acute vasodilator testing, and therefore, require therapy other than calcium channel antagonists. Children and adults treated with calcium channel blockers may lose this response over time and must be monitored carefully for sustained efficacy (see **Fig. 13**).[2,103]

PROSTACYCLINS

Adults with IPAH and children with CHD demonstrate an imbalance in the biosynthesis of thromboxane A_2 and prostacyclin.[104,105] Likewise, adults and children with severe PH show diminished prostacyclin synthase expression in the lung vasculature.[106] Prostacyclin administered over the long term, using intravenous epoprostenol, has been shown to improve survival and quality of life in adults and children with IPAH.[2,3,103,107–109]

Prostacyclin and prostacyclin analogues impact the cAMP pathway to increase pulmonary vasodilation. Intravenous epoprostenol-prostacyclin was

Table 1
Risk factors that should be considered when planning therapeutic management options in pulmonary hypertension

Lower Risk	Determinants of Risk	Higher Risk
No	Clinical evidence of RV failure	Yes
No	Progression of symptoms	Yes
No	Syncope	Yes
—	Growth	Failure to thrive
I, II	WHO-FC	III, IV
Minimally elevated	BNP/NT-proBNP	Significantly elevated Rising level
—	Echocardiography	Severe RV enlargement/dysfunction Pericardial effusion
Systemic CI >3.0 L/min/m² mPAP/mSAP <0.75 Acute vasoreactivity	Hemodynamics	Systemic CI <2.5 L/min/m² mPAP/mSAP >0.75 RAP >10 mm Hg PVRI >20 WU*m²

Abbreviations: CI, cardiac index; mPAP, mean pulmonary artery pressure; mSAP, mean systemic aortic pressure; RAP, right atrial pressure; SBNP, serum brain natriuretic peptide.
From Ivy DD, Abman SH, Barst RJ, et al. Pediatric pulmonary hypertension. J Am Coll Cardiol 2013;62(Suppl 25):D117–26; with permission.

first used in the 1980s and continues to be the gold standard for treatment of severe disease. Epoprostenol was US Food and Drug Administration (FDA) approved in 1995. Seventy-seven children diagnosed between 1982 and 1995 with IPAH were followed through 2002. Survival for all children treated with epoprostenol (n = 35) at 1, 5, and 10 years was 94%, 81%, and 61%, respectively, while treatment success was 83%, 57%, and 37%, respectively.[103] A more recent study of 77 children treated with epoprostenol or treprostinil showed a 5 year survival of 70% (**Fig. 14**).[107] The dose of intravenous prostacyclin in young children is usually higher than adults.

The prostacyclin analogue, treprostinil, was approved by the FDA, initially for subcutaneous use (2002), intravenous administration (2004), inhaled administration (2009), and oral treatment (2013). Although subcutaneous treprostinil allows patients to remain free of central venous catheters, it can cause severe pain at the infusion site. Long-term efficacy of subcutaneous treprostinil[110] and intravenous treprostinil[111] has been evaluated in adults with PAH. Intravenous treprostinil requires central line access and continuous infusion, but is easier for families to mix, may be used at room temperature, and has a half-life of 4 hours. Intravenous treprostinil has fewer side effects than intravenous epoprostenol, but there are no studies comparing efficacy.[112] Some studies have suggested a higher rate of bacteremia in children and adults treated with intravenous treprostinil,[113] but this may be decreased by protecting catheter connections and avoiding water on any connection.[114]

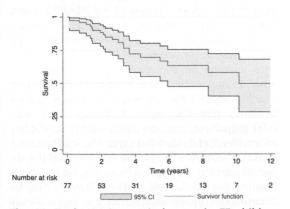

Fig. 14. Kaplan-Meier survival curve in 77 children with PH treated with epoprostenol or treprostinil, and those who transitioned, with 95% confidence intervals (CI) depicted. Transplant-free 5-year survival was 70% (95% CI, 56%–80%). (*From* Siehr SL, Ivy DD, Miller-Reed K, et al. Children with pulmonary arterial hypertension and prostanoid therapy: long-term hemodynamics. J Heart Lung Transplant 2013;32(5):546–52; with permission.)

Subcutaneous treprostinil in young children is well tolerated in many children with tolerable side effects.[115,116] Treprostinil has also been studied in an inhaled form.[117–119] Oral treprostinil was shown to effective as initial monotherapy treatment in adult PAH,[120] but not as add-on therapy.[121] Studies using oral treprostinil in children are ongoing.

Iloprost, an inhaled prostacyclin analogue, received approval for the treatment of PAH in the United States in December 2004. This medication is administered by nebulization 6 to 9 times a day. Iloprost requires patient cooperation with the treatment administration lasting 10 to 15 minutes,[122] which is difficult for young children.[123] In the acute setting, inhaled iloprost lowers mean pulmonary artery pressure and improves systemic oxygen saturation.[124] Some children may develop reactive airways obstruction limiting usefulness of this therapy. Selexipag, an oral selective IP prostacyclin-receptor agonist that is structurally distinct from prostacyclin, is approved for use in adults but has not been studied yet in children.

ENDOTHELIN RECEPTOR ANTAGONISTS

Another target for treatment of PH is the vasoconstrictor peptide ET.[125] The endothelins are a family of isopeptides consisting of ET-1, ET-2, and ET-3. ET-1 is a potent vasoactive peptide produced primarily in the vascular endothelial cell, but also may be produced by smooth muscle cells. Two receptor subtypes, ET_A and ET_B, mediate the activity of ET-1. ET_A and ET_B receptors on vascular smooth muscle mediate vasoconstriction, whereas ET_B receptors on endothelial cells cause release of NO and prostacyclin, and act as clearance receptors for circulating ET-1. ET-1 expression is increased in the pulmonary arteries of patients with PH.

Bosentan, a dual ET receptor antagonist, lowers pulmonary artery pressure and resistance and improves exercise tolerance in adults with PAH.[125] Bosentan has been approved since 2001 for the treatment of WHO-FC III and IV patients over 12 years of age and has recently shown beneficial effects in class II patients.[126] These results have been extrapolated to children.[109,127–134] Bosentan therapy added on to epoprostenol in children allowed for a decrease in epoprostenol dose and its associated side effects.[109] A more recent retrospective study of 86 children on bosentan for a median exposure of 14 months with and without concomitant therapy found that bosentan as part of an overall treatment strategy provided a sustained clinical and hemodynamic improvement that was overall well tolerated, and 2 year survival estimates were 91%. In this study, 90% improved or remained unchanged in WHO-FC after median treatment duration of 14 months.[133] Comparable results were reported by Maiya and colleagues,[132] except that in IPAH, stabilization was achieved in 95% but combined therapy with epoprostenol was necessary in 60%. Elevated hepatic aminotransferase levels occur in approximately 12% of adults treated with bosentan but were only 3.5% in children.[133] Recently, a European, prospective, noninterventional, Internet-based after-marketing surveillance database of bosentan was evaluated. Pediatric patients (aged 2–11 years) were compared with patients over 12 years of age. Over a 30-month period, 4994 patients, including 146 bosentan-naive pediatric patients, were captured in the database. PAH was idiopathic in 40% and related to CHD in 45%. The median exposure to bosentan was 29.1 weeks, and elevated aminotransferases were reported in 2.7% of children less than 12 years of age versus 7.8% in older patients. The discontinuation rate was 14.4% in children versus 28.1% in patients older than 12 years of age.[131] A pediatric formulation of bosentan is approved in Europe.[129] Macitentan, a dual ET-receptor antagonist, was FDA approved in 2013. Macitentan reduced the time from the initiation of treatment to the first occurrence of a composite end point of death, atrial septostomy, lung transplantation, initiation of treatment with intravenous, or subcutaneous prostanoids, or worsening of PAH.[135]

Selective ET$_A$ receptor blockade using ambrisentan may benefit patients with PAH by blocking the vasoconstrictor effects of ET$_A$ receptors while maintaining the vasodilator/clearance functions of ET$_B$ receptors. Ambrisentan was approved by the FDA in June 2007. Adults showed significant improvements in 6MW distance and significant delay in clinical worsening on ambrisentan. The incidence of elevated hepatic aminotransferase levels was 2.8%.[136] Initial experience with ambrisentan in children suggests that treatment is safe with similar pharmacokinetics to those in adults and may improve PAH in some children.[137,138]

PHOSPHODIESTERASE-5 INHIBITORS AND SOLUBLE GUANYLATE CYCLASE STIMULATORS

In models of PAH, phosphodiesterase-5 activity is increased and protein is localized to vascular smooth muscle.[139] Specific phosphodiesterase-5 inhibitors, such as sildenafil,[140,141] and tadalafil[142–145] promote an increase in cGMP levels and thus promote pulmonary vasodilation and remodeling. In certain settings, intravenous sildenafil may worsen oxygenation.[146,147] Sildenafil has been shown to prevent rebound PAH on withdrawal from inhaled NO.[148,149] Addition of sildenafil to long-term intravenous epoprostenol therapy in adults with PAH has been shown to be beneficial.[126]

Sildenafil has been approved for the treatment of WHO-FC II–IV PAH adult patients.[141] Sildenafil has been extensively studied in children with PAH.[140,150–153] In the 16-week, randomized, double-blind study, Sildenafil in Treatment-Naive Children, Aged 1 to 17 Years, With Pulmonary Arterial Hypertension (STARTS-1), the effects of oral sildenafil in pediatric PAH were studied.[154] Children (n = 235) with PAH (aged 1–17 years; ≥8 kg) received low-, medium-, or high-dose sildenafil or placebo orally 3 times daily. The trial did not meet its primary endpoint because estimated mean ± standard error percentage change in pVO$_2$ for the low, medium, and high doses combined versus placebo was 7.7% ± 4.0% (95% confidence interval, –0.2% to 15.6%; P = .056; see **Fig. 9**).[154] After the initial 16-week study, patients in the low-, medium-, and high-dose groups remained on that dose.[155] Patients in the placebo group were randomized to low, medium, or high dose; patients were then followed for the duration of the study. By 3 years, the hazard ratio for mortality was 3.95 (95% confidence interval, 1.46–10.65) for high versus low dose. Most patients who died had idiopathic/heritable PAH (76% vs 33% overall) and baseline FC III/IV disease (38% vs 15% overall); patients who died had worse baseline hemodynamics. Kaplan-Meier–estimated 3-year survival rates from the start of sildenafil were 94%, 93%, and 88% for patients randomized to low-, medium-, and high-dose sildenafil, respectively (**Fig. 15**). Based on this, the data monitoring committee recommended that all patients down-titrate from the high dose. Review of the STARTS-1 and -2 by the FDA and the European Medicines Agency (EMA) resulted in disparate recommendations. Sildenafil was approved by the EMA in 2011, with a later warning on avoidance of use of the high dose. In August 2012, the FDA released a strong warning against the (chronic) use of sildenafil for pediatric patients (ages 1 through 17) with PAH (http://www.fda.gov/Safety/MedWatch/Safety Information/SafetyAlertsforHumanMedicalProducts/ ucm317743.htm). In 2014, the FDA clarified the sildenafil warning, stating that there may be situations in which the risk-benefit profile of Revatio may be acceptable in individual children, and that sildenafil is still not recommended in children with PH (http:// www.fda.gov/Drugs/DrugSafety/ucm390876.htm).

Tadalalfil, another selective phosphodiesterase type 5 inhibitor, has a longer duration of action. In a study of 33 children with PAH, 29 were switched from sildenafil to tadalafil primarily for once-daily dosing. The average dose of sildenafil was 3.4 ± 1.1 mg/kg/d, and that of tadalafil

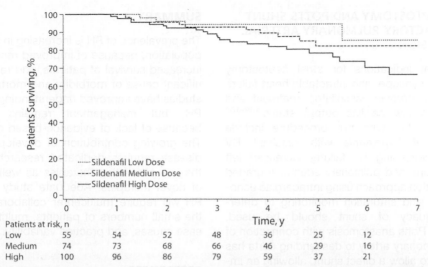

Fig. 15. Kaplan-Meier estimated survival from start of sildenafil treatment in STARTS-1 and STARTS-2 trials. Patients were censored at the last date they were known to be alive; if a patient received a transplant, he or she was censored the day before transplant. Patients at risk are those who are ongoing in the study or known to be alive at the specified time (ie, not dead, not lost to follow-up, or not in study long enough to reach time point). (*From* Barst RJ, Beghetti M, Pulido T, et al. STARTS-2: long-term survival with oral sildenafil monotherapy in treatment-naïve pediatric pulmonary arterial hypertension. Circulation 2014;129(19):1914–23; with permission.)

was 1.0 ± 0.4 mg/kg/d. For 14 of the 29 patients undergoing repeat catheterization, statistically significant improvements were observed after transition from sildenafil to tadalafil in terms of PAP and PVRI. Tadalafil was well tolerated, except in 2 children who discontinued for migraine or allergic reaction, and appeared to slow disease progression.[142]

Stimulation of the NO-cGMP pathway has revolutionized care of the patient with PH. Riociguat, a direct oral soluble sGC stimulator, increases cGMP directly in a non-NO-dependent manner but also increases the sensitivity of sGC to NO.[156] Riociguat was approved by the FDA in 2013 for the treatment of adult PAH[157] and is the first FDA-approved drug for the treatment of chronic thromboembolic PH.[158]

COMBINATION THERAPY

By targeting multiple pathways, combination therapy is appealing as treatment in more severe disease. Between 2000 and 2010, pediatric patients with PAH were compared between 3 centers. Treatment with PAH-targeted combination therapy during the study period was independently and strongly associated with improved survival compared with monotherapy (**Fig. 16**).[3]

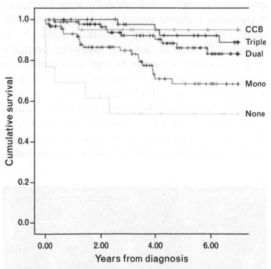

Fig. 16. Survival according to extent of PH therapy in 275 recently diagnosed consecutive pediatric PAH patients at 3 referral centers between 2000 and 2010. Survival improves on combination therapy for PH over monotherapy. (*From* Zijlstra WM, Douwes JM, Rosenzweig EB. Survival differences in pediatric pulmonary arterial hypertension: clues to a better understanding of outcome and optimal treatment strategies. J Am Coll Cardiol 2014;63(20):2159–69; with permission.)

ATRIAL SEPTOSTOMY AND POTTS SHUNT FOR REFRACTORY PULMONARY ARTERIAL HYPERTENSION

The general indications for atrial septostomy include PH, syncope, and intractable heart failure refractory to chronic vasodilator treatment and symptomatic low cardiac output states.[159–162] Risks associated with this procedure include worsening of hypoxemia with resultant RV ischemia, worsening RV failure, increased left atrial pressure, and pulmonary edema. A graded balloon dilation approach using intracardiac echocardiogram and saturation monitoring to determine adequacy of shunt should be used. Recently, a Potts anastomosis with connection of the left pulmonary artery to descending aorta has been used to allow a direct shunt, allowing an immediate reduction in RV afterload.[163–165] A Potts shunt may unload the right ventricle in systole, whereas an atrial septostomy provides a diastolic unloading. Treatment of right heart failure with the Potts shunt is increasing (**Fig. 17**).

TRANSPLANTATION

For patients who do not respond to prolonged vasodilator treatment, lung transplantation should be considered.[166–168] Cystic fibrosis accounts for most pediatric lung transplants. IPAH is the second most common indication for lung transplant in pediatric patients overall and is the most common indication among children aged 1 to 5 years.[169] Overall survival following pediatric lung transplant is similar to that encountered in adult patients, with recent registry data indicating a median survival of 4.9 years.[169–171] The most common causes of after-transplant death include graft failure, technical issues, and infection, whereas infection and bronchiolitis obliterans syndrome are the most common causes of late death.

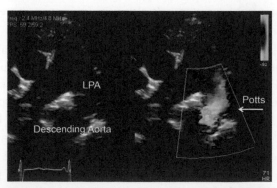

Fig. 17. Echocardiogram with color compare of the Potts shunt in a patient with severe IPAH. LPA, left pulmonary artery.

SUMMARY

The prevalence of PH is increasing in the pediatric population, because of improved recognition and increased survival of patients, and remains a significant cause of morbidity and mortality. Recent studies have improved understanding of pediatric PH, but management remains challenging because of lack of evidence-based clinical trials. The growing contribution of developmental lung disease requires dedicated research to explore the use of existing therapies as well as creation of novel therapies. Adequate study of pediatric PH will require multicenter collaboration due to the small numbers of patients, multifactorial disease causes, and practice variability.

REFERENCES

1. D'Alonzo GE, Barst RJ, Ayres SM, et al. Survival in patients with primary pulmonary hypertension. Results from a national prospective registry. Ann Intern Med 1991;115:343–9.
2. Barst RJ, Maislin G, Fishman AP. Vasodilator therapy for primary pulmonary hypertension in children. Circulation 1999;99:1197–208.
3. Zijlstra WM, Douwes JM, Rosenzweig EB, et al. Survival differences in pediatric pulmonary arterial hypertension: clues to a better understanding of outcome and optimal treatment strategies. J Am Coll Cardiol 2014;63:2159–69.
4. Ivy DD, Abman SH, Barst RJ, et al. Pediatric pulmonary hypertension. J Am Coll Cardiol 2013;62: D117–26.
5. Barst RJ, Ertel SI, Beghetti M, et al. Pulmonary arterial hypertension: a comparison between children and adults. Eur Respir J 2011;37:665–77.
6. Cerro MJ, Abman S, Diaz G, et al. A consensus approach to the classification of pediatric pulmonary hypertensive vascular disease: report from the PVRI Pediatric Taskforce, Panama 2011. Pulm Circ 2011;1:286–98.
7. Galie N, Corris PA, Frost A, et al. Updated treatment algorithm of pulmonary arterial hypertension. J Am Coll Cardiol 2013;62:D60–72.
8. Galie N, Humbert M, Vachiery JL, et al. 2015 ESC/ ERS guidelines for the diagnosis and treatment of pulmonary hypertension: the Joint Task Force for the Diagnosis and Treatment of Pulmonary Hypertension of the European Society of Cardiology (ESC) and the European Respiratory Society (ERS): endorsed by: Association for European Paediatric and Congenital Cardiology (AEPC), International Society for Heart and Lung Transplantation (ISHLT). Eur Respir J 2015;46(4):903–75.
9. Baruteau AE, Belli E, Boudjemline Y, et al. Palliative Potts shunt for the treatment of children with

drug-refractory pulmonary arterial hypertension: updated data from the first 24 patients. Eur J Cardiothorac Surg 2015;47:e105–10.

10. Hoeper MM, Bogaard HJ, Condliffe R, et al. Definitions and diagnosis of pulmonary hypertension. J Am Coll Cardiol 2013;62:D42–50.

11. Simonneau G, Gatzoulis MA, Adatia I, et al. Updated clinical classification of pulmonary hypertension. J Am Coll Cardiol 2013;62:D34–41.

12. Moledina S, Hislop AA, Foster H, et al. Childhood idiopathic pulmonary arterial hypertension: a national cohort study. Heart 2010;96:1401–6.

13. van Loon RL, Roofthooft MT, Hillege HL, et al. Pediatric pulmonary hypertension in the Netherlands: epidemiology and characterization during the period 1991 to 2005. Circulation 2011;124(16): 1755–64.

14. Cerro Marin MJ, Sabate Rotes A, Rodriguez Ogando A, et al. Assessing pulmonary hypertensive vascular disease in childhood: data from the Spanish registry. Am J Respir Crit Care Med 2014;190(12):1421–9.

15. Haworth SG, Hislop AA. Treatment and survival in children with pulmonary arterial hypertension: the UK Pulmonary Hypertension Service for Children 2001-2006. Heart 2009;95:312–7.

16. Maxwell BG, Nies MK, Ajuba-Iwuji CC, et al. Trends in hospitalization for pediatric pulmonary hypertension. Pediatrics 2015;136:241–50.

17. Frank DB, Crystal MA, Morales DL, et al. Trends in pediatric pulmonary hypertension-related hospitalizations in the United States from 2000-2009. Pulm Circ 2015;5:339–48.

18. Austin ED, Loyd JE. The genetics of pulmonary arterial hypertension. Circ Res 2014;115:189–202.

19. Soubrier F, Chung WK, Machado R, et al. Genetics and genomics of pulmonary arterial hypertension. J Am Coll Cardiol 2013;62:D13–21.

20. Rosenzweig EB, Morse JH, Knowles JA, et al. Clinical implications of determining BMPR2 mutation status in a large cohort of children and adults with pulmonary arterial hypertension. J Heart Lung Transpl 2008;27:668–74.

21. Harrison RE, Berger R, Haworth SG, et al. Transforming growth factor-beta receptor mutations and pulmonary arterial hypertension in childhood. Circulation 2005;111:435–41.

22. Lane KB, Machado RD, Pauciulo MW, et al. Heterozygous germline mutations in BMPR2, encoding a TGF-beta receptor, cause familial primary pulmonary hypertension. The International PPH Consortium. Nat Genet 2000;26:81–4.

23. Deng Z, Morse JH, Slager SL, et al. Familial primary pulmonary hypertension (gene PPH1) is caused by mutations in the bone morphogenetic protein receptor-II gene. Am J Hum Genet 2000; 67:737–44.

24. Grunig E, Koehler R, Miltenberger-Miltenyi G, et al. Primary pulmonary hypertension in children may have a different genetic background than in adults. Pediatr Res 2004;56:571–8.

25. Fujiwara M, Yagi H, Matsuoka R, et al. Implications of mutations of activin receptor-like kinase 1 gene (ALK1) in addition to bone morphogenetic protein receptor II gene (BMPR2) in children with pulmonary arterial hypertension. Circ J 2008;72:127–33.

26. Ma L, Chung WK. The genetic basis of pulmonary arterial hypertension. Hum Genet 2014;133: 471–9.

27. Best DH, Austin ED, Chung WK, et al. Genetics of pulmonary hypertension. Curr Opin Cardiol 2014; 29:520–7.

28. Kerstjens-Frederikse WS, Bongers EM, Roofthooft MT, et al. TBX4 mutations (small patella syndrome) are associated with childhood-onset pulmonary arterial hypertension. J Med Genet 2013;50:500–6.

29. La Gerche A, Gewillig M. What limits cardiac performance during exercise in normal subjects and in healthy Fontan patients? Int J Pediatr 2010; 2010 [pii:791291].

30. John AS, Johnson JA, Khan M, et al. Clinical outcomes and improved survival in patients with protein-losing enteropathy after the Fontan operation. J Am Coll Cardiol 2014;64:54–62.

31. Haseyama K, Satomi G, Yasukochi S, et al. Pulmonary vasodilation therapy with sildenafil citrate in a patient with plastic bronchitis after the Fontan procedure for hypoplastic left heart syndrome. J Thorac Cardiovasc Surg 2006;132:1232–3.

32. Malhotra SP, Ivy DD, Mitchell MB, et al. Performance of cavopulmonary palliation at elevated altitude: midterm outcomes and risk factors for failure. Circulation 2008;118:S177–81.

33. Levy M, Danel C, Laval AM, et al. Nitric oxide synthase expression by pulmonary arteries: a predictive marker of Fontan procedure outcome? J Thorac Cardiovasc Surg 2003;125:1083–90.

34. Mitchell MB, Campbell DN, Ivy D, et al. Evidence of pulmonary vascular disease after heart transplantation for Fontan circulation failure. J Thorac Cardiovasc Surg 2004;128:693–702.

35. Van De Bruaene A, La Gerche A, Claessen G, et al. Sildenafil improves exercise hemodynamics in Fontan patients. Circ Cardiovasc Imaging 2014;7:265–73.

36. Goldberg DJ, French B, Szwast AL, et al. Impact of sildenafil on echocardiographic indices of myocardial performance after the Fontan operation. Pediatr Cardiol 2012;33:689–96.

37. Morchi GS, Ivy DD, Duster MC, et al. Sildenafil increases systemic saturation and reduces pulmonary artery pressure in patients with failing fontan physiology. Congenit Heart Dis 2009;4:107–11.

38. Yamagishi M, Kurosawa H, Hashimoto K, et al. The role of plasma endothelin in the Fontan circulation. J Cardiovasc Surg (torino) 2002;43:793–7.

39. Hebert A, Mikkelsen UR, Thilen U, et al. Bosentan improves exercise capacity in adolescents and adults after Fontan operation: the TEMPO (treatment with endothelin receptor antagonist in Fontan patients, a randomized, placebo-controlled, double-blind study measuring peak oxygen consumption) study. Circulation 2014;130:2021–30.

40. Derk G, Houser L, Miner P, et al. Efficacy of endothelin blockade in adults with Fontan physiology. Congenit Heart Dis 2015;10(1):E11–6.

41. Bowater SE, Weaver RA, Thorne SA, et al. The safety and effects of bosentan in patients with a Fontan circulation. Congenit Heart Dis 2012;7:243–9.

42. Krishnan U, Rosenzweig EB. Pulmonary hypertension in chronic lung disease of infancy. Curr Opin Pediatr 2015;27:177–83.

43. Mourani PM, Sontag MK, Younoszai A, et al. Early pulmonary vascular disease in preterm infants at risk for bronchopulmonary dysplasia. Am J Respir Crit Care Med 2015;191:87–95.

44. Abman SH, Hansmann G, Archer SL, et al. Pediatric pulmonary hypertension: guidelines from the American Heart Association and American Thoracic Society. Circulation 2015;132(21):2037–99.

45. del Cerro MJ, Sabate Rotes A, Carton A, et al. Pulmonary hypertension in bronchopulmonary dysplasia: clinical findings, cardiovascular anomalies and outcomes. Pediatr Pulmonol 2014;49:49–59.

46. Khemani E, McElhinney DB, Rhein L, et al. Pulmonary artery hypertension in formerly premature infants with bronchopulmonary dysplasia: clinical features and outcomes in the surfactant era. Pediatrics 2007;120:1260–9.

47. Beghetti M, Berger RM, Schulze-Neick I, et al. Diagnostic evaluation of paediatric pulmonary hypertension in current clinical practice. Eur Respir J 2013;42:689–700.

48. Jone PN, Ivy DD. Echocardiography in pediatric pulmonary hypertension. Front Pediatr 2014;2:124.

49. Forfia PR, Fisher MR, Mathai SC, et al. Tricuspid annular displacement predicts survival in pulmonary hypertension. Am J Respir Crit Care Med 2006;174:1034–41.

50. Galie N, Hinderliter AL, Torbicki A, et al. Effects of the oral endothelin-receptor antagonist bosentan on echocardiographic and Doppler measures in patients with pulmonary arterial hypertension. J Am Coll Cardiol 2003;41:1380–6.

51. Hinderliter AL, Willis PW, Barst RJ, et al. Effects of long-term infusion of prostacyclin (epoprostenol) on echocardiographic measures of right ventricular structure and function in primary pulmonary hypertension. Primary Pulmonary Hypertension Study Group. Circulation 1997;95:1479–86.

52. Koestenberger M, Ravekes W, Everett AD, et al. Right ventricular function in infants, children and adolescents: reference values of the tricuspid annular plane systolic excursion (TAPSE) in 640 healthy patients and calculation of z score values. J Am Soc Echocardiogr 2009;22:715–9.

53. Raymond RJ, Hinderliter AL, Willis PW, et al. Echocardiographic predictors of adverse outcomes in primary pulmonary hypertension. J Am Coll Cardiol 2002;39:1214–9.

54. Tei C, Dujardin KS, Hodge DO, et al. Doppler echocardiographic index for assessment of global right ventricular function. J Am Soc Echocardiography 1996;9:838–47.

55. Dyer KL, Pauliks LB, Das B, et al. Use of myocardial performance index in pediatric patients with idiopathic pulmonary arterial hypertension. J Am Soc Echocardiogr 2006;19:21–7.

56. Kassem E, Humpl T, Friedberg MK. Prognostic significance of 2-dimensional, M-mode, and Doppler echo indices of right ventricular function in children with pulmonary arterial hypertension. Am Heart J 2013;165:1024–31.

57. Jone PN, Hinzman J, Wagner BD, et al. Right ventricular to left ventricular diameter ratio at end-systole in evaluating outcomes in children with pulmonary hypertension. J Am Soc Echocardiogr 2014;27:172–8.

58. Masuyama T, Kodama K, Kitabatake A, et al. Continuous-wave Doppler echocardiographic detection of pulmonary regurgitation and its application to noninvasive estimation of pulmonary artery pressure. Circulation 1986;74:484–92.

59. Benza RL, Miller DP, Gomberg-Maitland M, et al. Predicting survival in pulmonary arterial hypertension: insights from the registry to evaluate early and long-term pulmonary arterial hypertension disease management (REVEAL). Circulation 2010;122:164–72.

60. Alkon J, Humpl T, Manlhiot C, et al. Usefulness of the right ventricular systolic to diastolic duration ratio to predict functional capacity and survival in children with pulmonary arterial hypertension. Am J Cardiol 2010;106:430–6.

61. Friedberg MK, Redington AN. Right versus left ventricular failure: differences, similarities, and interactions. Circulation 2014;129:1033–44.

62. Lammers AE, Haworth SG, Riley G, et al. Value of tissue Doppler echocardiography in children with pulmonary hypertension. J Am Soc Echocardiogr 2012;25:504–10.

63. Takatsuki S, Nakayama T, Jone PN, et al. Tissue Doppler imaging predicts adverse outcome in children with idiopathic pulmonary arterial hypertension. J Pediatr 2012;161:1126–31.

64. Ozawa K, Funabashi N, Takaoka H, et al. Utility of three-dimensional global longitudinal strain of

the right ventricle using transthoracic echocardiography for right ventricular systolic function in pulmonary hypertension. Int J Cardiol 2014;174: 426–30.

65. Lu X, Nadvoretskiy V, Bu L, et al. Accuracy and reproducibility of real-time three-dimensional echocardiography for assessment of right ventricular volumes and ejection fraction in children. J Am Soc Echocardiogr 2008;21:84–9.

66. Geiger R, Strasak A, Treml B, et al. Six-minute walk test in children and adolescents. J Pediatr 2007; 150:395–9, 9.e1–2.

67. Lammers AE, Hislop AA, Flynn Y, et al. The 6-minute walk test: normal values for children of 4-11 years of age. Arch Dis Child 2008;93:464–8.

68. Lesser DJ, Fleming MM, Maher CA, et al. Does the 6-min walk test correlate with the exercise stress test in children? Pediatr pulmonology 2010;45:135–40.

69. Li AM, Yin J, Au JT, et al. Standard reference for the six-minute-walk test in healthy children aged 7 to 16 years. Am J Respir Crit Care Med 2007;176:174–80.

70. van Loon RL, Roofthooft MT, Delhaas T, et al. Outcome of pediatric patients with pulmonary arterial hypertension in the era of new medical therapies. Am J Cardiol 2010;106:117–24.

71. Garofano RP, Barst RJ. Exercise testing in children with primary pulmonary hypertension. Pediatr Cardiol 1999;20:61–4 [discussion: 65].

72. Yetman AT, Taylor AL, Doran A, et al. Utility of cardiopulmonary stress testing in assessing disease severity in children with pulmonary arterial hypertension. Am J Cardiol 2005;95:697–9.

73. Rausch CM, Taylor AL, Ross H, et al. Ventilatory efficiency slope correlates with functional capacity, outcomes, and disease severity in pediatric patients with pulmonary hypertension. Int J Cardiol 2013;169:445–8.

74. Nagaya N, Nishikimi T, Uematsu M, et al. Plasma brain natriuretic peptide as a prognostic indicator in patients with primary pulmonary hypertension. Circulation 2000;102:865–70.

75. Lammers AE, Hislop AA, Haworth SG. Prognostic value of B-type natriuretic peptide in children with pulmonary hypertension. Int J Cardiol 2009;135: 21–6.

76. Bernus A, Wagner BD, Accurso F, et al. Brain natriuretic peptide levels in managing pediatric patients with pulmonary arterial hypertension. Chest 2009;135:745–51.

77. Van Albada ME, Loot FG, Fokkema R, et al. Biological serum markers in the management of pediatric pulmonary arterial hypertension. Pediatr Res 2008; 63:321–7.

78. Ploegstra MJ, Douwes JM, Roofthooft MT, et al. Identification of treatment goals in paediatric pulmonary arterial hypertension. Eur Respir J 2014; 44(6):1616–26.

79. Su Z, Tan W, Shandas R, et al. Influence of distal resistance and proximal stiffness on hemodynamics and RV afterload in progression and treatments of pulmonary hypertension: a computational study with validation using animal models. Comput Math Methods Med 2013;2013: 618326.

80. Su Z, Hunter KS, Shandas R. Impact of pulmonary vascular stiffness and vasodilator treatment in pediatric pulmonary hypertension: 21 patient-specific fluid-structure interaction studies. Computer Methods Programs Biomed 2012;108:617–28.

81. Hunter KS, Feinstein JA, Ivy DD, et al. Computational simulation of the pulmonary arteries and its role in the study of pediatric pulmonary hypertension. Prog Pediatr Cardiol 2010;30:63–9.

82. Friedberg MK, Feinstein JA, Rosenthal DN. Noninvasive assessment of pulmonary arterial capacitance by echocardiography. J Am Soc Echocardiogr 2007;20:186–90.

83. Douwes JM, Roofthooft MT, Bartelds B, et al. Pulsatile haemodynamic parameters are predictors of survival in paediatric pulmonary arterial hypertension. Int J Cardiol 2013;168:1370–7.

84. Di Maria MV, Younoszai AK, Mertens L, et al. RV stroke work in children with pulmonary arterial hypertension: estimation based on invasive haemodynamic assessment and correlation with outcomes. Heart 2014;100:1342–7.

85. Di Maria MV, Burkett DA, Younoszai AK, et al. Echocardiographic estimation of right ventricular stroke work in children with pulmonary arterial hypertension: comparison with invasive measurements. J Am Soc Echocardiogr 2015;28(11):1350–7.

86. Moledina S, Pandya B, Bartsota M, et al. Prognostic significance of cardiac magnetic resonance imaging in children with pulmonary hypertension. Circ Cardiovasc Imaging 2013;6:407–14.

87. Hall S, Brogan P, Haworth SG, et al. Contribution of inflammation to the pathology of idiopathic pulmonary arterial hypertension in children. Thorax 2009;64:778–83.

88. Nies MK, Ivy DD, Everett AD. The untapped potential of proteomic analysis in pediatric pulmonary hypertension. Proteomics Clin Appl 2014;8(11–12): 862–74.

89. Yeager ME, Colvin KL, Everett AD, et al. Plasma proteomics of differential outcome to long-term therapy in children with idiopathic pulmonary arterial hypertension. Proteomics Clin Appl 2012;6: 257–67.

90. Duncan M, Wagner BD, Murray K, et al. Circulating cytokines and growth factors in pediatric pulmonary hypertension. Mediators Inflamm 2012;2012: 143428.

91. Yeager ME, Nguyen CM, Belchenko DD, et al. Circulating myeloid-derived suppressor cells are

increased and activated in pulmonary hypertension. Chest 2012;141:944–52.

92. Sharma S, Umar S, Potus F, et al. Apolipoprotein A-I mimetic peptide 4F rescues pulmonary hypertension by inducing microRNA-193-3p. Circulation 2014;130:776–85.

93. Wagner BD, Takatsuki S, Accurso FJ, et al. Evaluation of circulating proteins and hemodynamics towards predicting mortality in children with pulmonary arterial hypertension. PLoS One 2013;8:e80235.

94. Olsson KM, Delcroix M, Ghofrani HA, et al. Anticoagulation and survival in pulmonary arterial hypertension: results from the comparative, prospective registry of newly initiated therapies for pulmonary hypertension (COMPERA). Circulation 2014;129:57–65.

95. Barst RJ, Abenhaim L. Fatal pulmonary arterial hypertension associated with phenylpropanolamine exposure. Heart 2004;90:e42.

96. Friesen RH, Williams GD. Anesthetic management of children with pulmonary arterial hypertension. Paediatr Anaesth 2008;18:208–16.

97. Carmosino MJ, Friesen RH, Doran A, et al. Perioperative complications in children with pulmonary hypertension undergoing noncardiac surgery or cardiac catheterization. Anesth Analg 2007;104:521–7.

98. Berman Rosenzweig E, Barst RJ. Pulmonary arterial hypertension: a comprehensive review of pharmacological treatment. Treat Respir Med 2006;5:117–27.

99. Beghetti M. Current treatment options in children with pulmonary arterial hypertension and experiences with oral bosentan. Eur J Clin Invest 2006;36(Suppl 3):16–24.

100. Douwes JM, van Loon RL, Hoendermis ES, et al. Acute pulmonary vasodilator response in paediatric and adult pulmonary arterial hypertension: occurrence and prognostic value when comparing three response criteria. Eur Heart J 2011;32(24):3137–46.

101. Sitbon O, Humbert M, Jais X, et al. Long-term response to calcium channel blockers in idiopathic pulmonary arterial hypertension. Circulation 2005;111:3105–11.

102. Barst RJ, McGoon MD, Elliott CG, et al. Survival in childhood pulmonary arterial hypertension: insights from the registry to evaluate early and long-term pulmonary arterial hypertension disease management. Circulation 2012;125:113–22.

103. Yung D, Widlitz AC, Rosenzweig EB, et al. Outcomes in children with idiopathic pulmonary arterial hypertension. Circulation 2004;110:660–5.

104. Christman BW, McPherson CD, Newman JH, et al. An imbalance between the excretion of thromboxane and prostacyclin metabolites in pulmonary hypertension. New Engl J Med 1992;327:70–5.

105. Adatia I, Barrow SE, Stratton PD, et al. Thromboxane A2 and prostacyclin biosynthesis in children and adolescents with pulmonary vascular disease. Circulation 1993;88:2117–22.

106. Tuder RM, Cool CD, Geraci MW, et al. Prostacyclin synthase expression is decreased in lungs from patients with severe pulmonary hypertension. Am J Respir Crit Care Med 1999;159:1925–32.

107. Siehr SL, Ivy DD, Miller-Reed K, et al. Children with pulmonary arterial hypertension and prostanoid therapy: long-term hemodynamics. J Heart Lung Transpl 2013;32:546–52.

108. Lammers AE, Hislop AA, Flynn Y, et al. Epoprostenol treatment in children with severe pulmonary hypertension. Heart 2007;93:739–43.

109. Ivy DD, Doran A, Claussen L, et al. Weaning and discontinuation of epoprostenol in children with idiopathic pulmonary arterial hypertension receiving concomitant bosentan. Am J Cardiol 2004;93:943–6.

110. Barst RJ, Galie N, Naeije R, et al. Long-term outcome in pulmonary arterial hypertension patients treated with subcutaneous treprostinil. Eur Respir J 2006;28:1195–203.

111. Gomberg-Maitland M, Tapson VF, Benza RL, et al. Transition from intravenous epoprostenol to intravenous treprostinil in pulmonary hypertension. Am J Respir Crit Care Med 2005;172:1586–9.

112. Ivy DD, Claussen L, Doran A. Transition of stable pediatric patients with pulmonary arterial hypertension from intravenous epoprostenol to intravenous treprostinil. Am J Cardiol 2007;99:696–8.

113. Centers for Disease Control and Prevention (CDC). Bloodstream infections among patients treated with intravenous epoprostenol or intravenous treprostinil for pulmonary arterial hypertension–seven sites, United States, 2003-2006. MMWR Morb Mortal Wkly Rep 2007;56:170–2.

114. Doran AK, Ivy DD, Barst RJ, et al. Guidelines for the prevention of central venous catheter-related blood stream infections with prostanoid therapy for pulmonary arterial hypertension. Int J Clin Pract Suppl 2008;(160):5–9.

115. Ferdman DJ, Rosenzweig EB, Zuckerman WA, et al. Subcutaneous treprostinil for pulmonary hypertension in chronic lung disease of infancy. Pediatrics 2014;134:e274–8.

116. Levy M, Celermajer DS, Bourges-Petit E, et al. Add-on therapy with subcutaneous treprostinil for refractory pediatric pulmonary hypertension. The J Pediatr 2011;158:584–8.

117. Takatsuki S, Parker DK, Doran AK, et al. Acute pulmonary vasodilator testing with inhaled treprostinil in children with pulmonary arterial hypertension. Pediatr Cardiol 2013;34:1006–12.

118. Krishnan U, Takatsuki S, Ivy DD, et al. Effectiveness and safety of inhaled treprostinil for the treatment of

pulmonary arterial hypertension in children. Am J Cardiol 2012;110:1704–9.

119. Voswinckel R, Enke B, Reichenberger F, et al. Favorable effects of inhaled treprostinil in severe pulmonary hypertension: results from randomized controlled pilot studies. J Am Coll Cardiol 2006; 48:1672–81.

120. Jing ZC, Parikh K, Pulido T, et al. Efficacy and safety of oral treprostinil monotherapy for the treatment of pulmonary arterial hypertension: a randomized, controlled trial. Circulation 2013;127:624–33.

121. Tapson VF, Jing ZC, Xu KF, et al. Oral treprostinil for the treatment of pulmonary arterial hypertension in patients receiving background endothelin receptor antagonist and phosphodiesterase type 5 inhibitor therapy (the FREEDOM-C2 study): a randomized controlled trial. Chest 2013;144:952–8.

122. Olschewski H, Simonneau G, Galie N, et al. Inhaled iloprost for severe pulmonary hypertension. N Engl J Med 2002;347:322–9.

123. Ivy DD, Doran AK, Smith KJ, et al. Short- and long-term effects of inhaled iloprost therapy in children with pulmonary arterial hypertension. J Am Coll Cardiol 2008;51:161–9.

124. Limsuwan A, Wanitkul S, Khosithset A, et al. Aerosolized iloprost for postoperative pulmonary hypertensive crisis in children with congenital heart disease. Int J Cardiol 2008;129:333–8.

125. Rubin LJ, Badesch DB, Barst RJ, et al. Bosentan therapy for pulmonary arterial hypertension. N Engl J Med 2002;346:896–903.

126. Simonneau G, Rubin LJ, Galie N, et al. Addition of sildenafil to long-term intravenous epoprostenol therapy in patients with pulmonary arterial hypertension: a randomized trial. Ann Intern Med 2008; 149:521–30.

127. Taguchi M, Ichida F, Hirono K, et al. Pharmacokinetics of bosentan in routinely treated Japanese pediatric patients with pulmonary arterial hypertension. Drug Metab Pharmacokinet 2011;26(3):280–7.

128. Hislop AA, Moledina S, Foster H, et al. Long-term efficacy of bosentan in treatment of pulmonary arterial hypertension in children. Eur Respir J 2011;38:70–7.

129. Beghetti M, Haworth SG, Bonnet D, et al. Pharmacokinetic and clinical profile of a novel formulation of bosentan in children with pulmonary arterial hypertension: the FUTURE-1 study. Br J Clin Pharmacol 2009;68:948–55.

130. Beghetti M. Bosentan in pediatric patients with pulmonary arterial hypertension. Curr Vasc Pharmacol 2009;7:225–33.

131. Beghetti M, Hoeper MM, Kiely DG, et al. Safety experience with bosentan in 146 children 2-11 years old with pulmonary arterial hypertension: results from the European Postmarketing Surveillance program. Pediatr Res 2008;64:200–4.

132. Maiya S, Hislop AA, Flynn Y, et al. Response to bosentan in children with pulmonary hypertension. Heart 2006;92:664–70.

133. Rosenzweig EB, Ivy DD, Widlitz A, et al. Effects of long-term bosentan in children with pulmonary arterial hypertension. J Am Coll Cardiol 2005;46: 697–704.

134. Barst RJ, Ivy D, Dingemanse J, et al. Pharmacokinetics, safety, and efficacy of bosentan in pediatric patients with pulmonary arterial hypertension. Clin Pharmacol Ther 2003;73:372–82.

135. Pulido T, Adzerikho I, Channick RN, et al. Macitentan and morbidity and mortality in pulmonary arterial hypertension. N Engl J Med 2013;369:809–18.

136. Galie N, Olschewski H, Oudiz RJ, et al. Ambrisentan for the treatment of pulmonary arterial hypertension: results of the ambrisentan in pulmonary arterial hypertension, randomized, double-blind, placebo-controlled, multicenter, efficacy (ARIES) study 1 and 2. Circulation 2008;117:3010–9.

137. Takatsuki S, Rosenzweig EB, Zuckerman W, et al. Clinical safety, pharmacokinetics, and efficacy of ambrisentan therapy in children with pulmonary arterial hypertension. Pediatr Pulmonol 2013;48: 27–34.

138. Zuckerman WA, Leaderer D, Rowan CA, et al. Ambrisentan for pulmonary arterial hypertension due to congenital heart disease. Am J Cardiol 2011; 107:1381–5.

139. Hanson KA, Ziegler JW, Rybalkin SD, et al. Chronic pulmonary hypertension increases fetal lung cGMP phosphodiesterase activity. Am J Physiol 1998; 275:L931–41.

140. Humpl T, Reyes JT, Holtby H, et al. Beneficial effect of oral sildenafil therapy on childhood pulmonary arterial hypertension: twelve-month clinical trial of a single-drug, open-label, pilot study. Circulation 2005;111:3274–80.

141. Galie N, Ghofrani HA, Torbicki A, et al. Sildenafil citrate therapy for pulmonary arterial hypertension. N Engl J Med 2005;353:2148–57.

142. Takatsuki S, Calderbank M, Ivy DD. Initial experience with tadalafil in pediatric pulmonary arterial hypertension. Pediatr Cardiol 2012;33:683–8.

143. Pettit RS, Johnson CE, Caruthers RL. Stability of an extemporaneously prepared tadalafil suspension. Am J health-system Pharm 2012;69:592–4.

144. Rosenzweig EB. Tadalafil for the treatment of pulmonary arterial hypertension. Expert Opin Pharmacother 2010;11:127–32.

145. Galie N, Brundage BH, Ghofrani HA, et al. Tadalafil therapy for pulmonary arterial hypertension. Circulation 2009;119:2894–903.

146. Schulze-Neick I, Hartenstein P, Li J, et al. Intravenous sildenafil is a potent pulmonary vasodilator in children with congenital heart disease. Circulation 2003;108(Suppl 1):II167–73.

147. Stocker C, Penny DJ, Brizard CP, et al. Intravenous sildenafil and inhaled nitric oxide: a randomised trial in infants after cardiac surgery. Intensive Care Med 2003;29:1996–2003.

148. Atz AM, Wessel DL. Sildenafil ameliorates effects of inhaled nitric oxide withdrawal. Anesthesiology 1999;91:307–10.

149. Namachivayam P, Theilen U, Butt WW, et al. Sildenafil prevents rebound pulmonary hypertension after withdrawal of nitric oxide in children. Am J Respir Crit Care Med 2006;174:1042–7.

150. Karatza AA, Bush A, Magee AG. Safety and efficacy of sildenafil therapy in children with pulmonary hypertension. Int J Cardiol 2005;100:267–73.

151. Fasnacht MS, Tolsa JF, Beghetti M. The Swiss registry for pulmonary arterial hypertension: the paediatric experience. Swiss Med Wkly 2007;137:510–3.

152. Mourani PM, Sontag MK, Ivy DD, et al. Effects of long-term sildenafil treatment for pulmonary hypertension in infants with chronic lung disease. J Pediatr 2009;154:379–84, 84.e1–2.

153. Haworth SG. The management of pulmonary hypertension in children. Arch Dis Child 2008;93:620–5.

154. Barst RJ, Ivy DD, Gaitan G, et al. A randomized, double-blind, placebo-controlled, dose-ranging study of oral sildenafil citrate in treatment-naive children with pulmonary arterial hypertension. Circulation 2012;125:324–34.

155. Barst RJ, Beghetti M, Pulido T, et al. STARTS-2: long-term survival with oral Sildenafil monotherapy in treatment-naive pediatric pulmonary arterial hypertension. Circulation 2014;129:1914–23.

156. Schermuly RT, Janssen W, Weissmann N, et al. Riociguat for the treatment of pulmonary hypertension. Expert Opin Investig Drugs 2011;20:567–76.

157. Ghofrani HA, Galie N, Grimminger F, et al. Riociguat for the treatment of pulmonary arterial hypertension. N Engl J Med 2013;369:330–40.

158. Ghofrani HA, D'Armini AM, Grimminger F, et al. Riociguat for the treatment of chronic thromboembolic pulmonary hypertension. N Engl J Med 2013;369:319–29.

159. Barst RJ. Role of atrial septostomy in the treatment of pulmonary vascular disease. Thorax 2000;55:95–6.

160. Kerstein D, Levy PS, Hsu DT, et al. Blade balloon atrial septostomy in patients with severe primary pulmonary hypertension. Circulation 1995;91:2028–35.

161. Nihill MR, O'Laughlin MP, Mullins CE. Effects of atrial septostomy in patients with terminal cor pulmonale due to pulmonary vascular disease. Cathet Cardiovasc Diagn 1991;24:166–72.

162. Sandoval J, Gaspar J, Pulido T, et al. Graded balloon dilation atrial septostomy in severe primary pulmonary hypertension. A therapeutic alternative for patients nonresponsive to vasodilator treatment. J Am Coll Cardiol 1998;32:297–304.

163. Baruteau AE, Serraf A, Levy M, et al. Potts shunt in children with idiopathic pulmonary arterial hypertension: long-term results. Ann Thorac Surg 2012;94:817–24.

164. Labombarda F, Maragnes P, Dupont-Chauvet P, et al. Potts anastomosis for children with idiopathic pulmonary hypertension. Pediatr Cardiol 2009;30(8):1143–5.

165. Blanc J, Vouhe P, Bonnet D. Potts shunt in patients with pulmonary hypertension. N Engl J Med 2004;350:623.

166. Mallory GB, Spray TL. Paediatric lung transplantation. Eur Resp J 2004;24:839–45.

167. Toyoda Y, Thacker J, Santos R, et al. Long-term outcome of lung and heart-lung transplantation for idiopathic pulmonary arterial hypertension. Ann Thorac Surg 2008;86:1116–22.

168. Aurora P, Boucek MM, Christie J, et al. Registry of the International Society for Heart and Lung Transplantation: tenth official pediatric lung and heart/lung transplantation report–2007. J Heart Lung Transpl 2007;26:1223–8.

169. Kirkby S, Hayes D Jr. Pediatric lung transplantation: indications and outcomes. J Thorac Dis 2014;6:1024–31.

170. Khan MS, Heinle JS, Samayoa AX, et al. Is lung transplantation survival better in infants? Analysis of over 80 infants. J Heart Lung Transpl 2013;32:44–9.

171. Benden C, Edwards LB, Kucheryavaya AY, et al. The registry of the International Society for Heart and Lung Transplantation: sixteenth official pediatric lung and heart-lung transplantation Report–2013; focus theme: age. J Heart Lung Transpl 2013;32:989–97.

172. Mourani PM, Abman SH. Pulmonary vascular disease in bronchopulmonary dysplasia: pulmonary hypertension and beyond. Curr Opin Pediatr 2013;25(3):329–37.

173. An HS, Bae EJ, Kim GB. Pulmonary hypertension in preterm infants with bronchopulmonary dysplasia. Korean Circ J 2010;40(3):131–6.

174. Bhat R, Salas AA, Foster C. Prospective analysis of pulmonary hypertension in extremely low birth weight infants. Pediatrics 2012;129(3):e682–9.

Special Situations in Pulmonary Hypertension
Pregnancy and Right Ventricular Failure

Jana Svetlichnaya, MD, MSc*, Munir Janmohammed, MD,
Teresa De Marco, MD

KEYWORDS

- Pregnancy • Pulmonary arterial hypertension • Pulmonary vascular disease
- Right ventricular failure

KEY POINTS

- Pregnancy remains a high-risk hemodynamic state for patients with PAH despite some improvement in outcomes with the advent of modern PAH therapies and multidisciplinary management strategies.
- Right ventricular (RV) failure predicts a poor prognosis in patients with pulmonary arterial hypertension (PAH).
- Evidence-based therapy for PAH should be initiated early in the disease course to decrease RV wall stress and prevent RV remodeling and fibrosis.
- In patients with acutely decompensated RV failure, an aggressive and multifaceted approach must be used with a combination of oxygen, intravenous (IV), or inhaled pulmonary vasodilators; inotropic agents; and diuretics; a thorough search for triggering factors for the decompensation is a key part of the successful management strategy.
- At specialized centers, atrial septostomy, extracorporeal membrane oxygenation (ECMO), and mechanical circulatory support devices are options to bridge patients to lung or heart-lung transplantation.
- Patients with refractory RV failure who are not candidates for surgical intervention should be referred to palliative care to maximize quality of life and symptom relief.

PREGNANCY
Introduction

PAH frequently affects women of childbearing age. Pregnancy is known to be associated with a high incidence of maternal and fetal mortality and morbidity in patients with PAH: the largest systematic review to date reported a maternal mortality of 30% to 56% and neonatal mortality of 11% to 13% in patients with PAH.[1] The hemodynamic stressors of pregnancy can sometimes lead to a new diagnosis of PAH in previously asymptomatic women. Current guidelines recommend strict avoidance of pregnancy and early pregnancy termination in women with PAH.[2] The treatment of PAH has been revolutionized, however, in the past 2 decades with new classes of medications,

including endothelin receptor antagonists (ERAs), phosphodiesterase (PDE)-5 inhibitors, soluble guanyl cyclase stimulator, and prostacyclin analogs, resulting in dramatic improvement in quality of life, functional status, and, with epoprostenol, mortality outcomes. This article reviews the physiology of pregnancy in women with PAH and the therapeutic options and treatment outcomes in pregnancy in the modern era of PAH therapy.

Hemodynamic Effects of Pregnancy

Gestation: a hyperdynamic and hypercoagulable state

Progressive expansion of plasma volume is one of the physiologic hallmarks of pregnancy. Plasma volume expansion begins at 6 to 8 weeks'

Division of Cardiology, Department of Medicine, University of California San Francisco, San Francisco, CA, USA
* Corresponding author.
E-mail address: Jana.Svetlichnaya@ucsf.edu

Cardiol Clin 34 (2016) 473–487
http://dx.doi.org/10.1016/j.ccl.2016.04.007

gestation and increases by 50% during an average pregnancy to reach a peak intravascular volume of 4700 mL to 5200 mL at 32 weeks.[1,2] The resultant increase in stroke volume (SV) and a smaller-magnitude increase in resting heart rate (10–20 beats per minute) combine to increase cardiac output (CO) by 35% to a maximum of 9 L/min at term.[1,3] The highly compliant pulmonary vasculature of a healthy young woman coupled with further progesterone-mediated reduction in pulmonary vascular resistance (PVR) is able to accept this high CO without a rise in pulmonary pressure; in women with PAH, the vasoconstricted, remodeled pulmonary vasculature cannot respond with fall in PVR and there is a paradoxic increase in pulmonary pressures.[2] The dangerous combination of increased CO and elevated PVR presents a pressure overload to the RV with attendant high incidence of acute RV failure and maternal mortality during the peripartum, intrapartum, and postpartum periods in pregnant women with PAH.

Pregnancy is associated with a markedly hypercoagulable state due to increased fibrin generation, decreased fibrinolytic activity, increased levels of clotting factors, decrease in free protein S, and a high incidence of acquired resistance to protein C. These risk factors for thromboembolism are further exacerbated by a 50% reduction of venous flow velocity in the lower extremities due to compression by the enlarged uterus starting at 25 to 29 weeks' gestation and lasting until 6 weeks postdelivery.[4] These changes combine to raise the overall risk of thromboembolic events 5-fold in a pregnant woman even in the absence of PAH[5] but no data currently exist to quantify the precise incremental risk to pregnant women with PAH.

Peripartum and postpartum: a time of rapid hemodynamic shifts

The peripartum state is a time of large-scale volume shifts and rapid fluctuations in CO that poses further stress the RV in patients with PAH. In late gestation, the gravid uterus can compress the inferior vena cava, resulting in rapid decreases in venous return and drastic changes in preload to the RV merely with positional changes. Vaginal delivery is associated with blood loss of approximately 500 mL, or 10% loss of total blood volume, whereas caesarean section can amount to as much as 1000 mL, or up to 30% total plasma volume blood loss.[4] Uterine smooth muscle contraction postdelivery results in a rapid infusion of 300 mL to 500 mL of blood from the uterus into the maternal circulation.[6] Uterine contraction, anxiety, and pain also cause further increases in heart rate and thus CO during labor.[5]

The hemodynamic changes of pregnancy persist in the immediate postpartum period making this time one of the most dangerous in the course of pregnancy. There is a rapid increase in both systemic vascular resistance (SVR) and PVR that occurs immediately after delivery. The relief of compression of the inferior vena cava by the gravid uterus can result in rapid preload increase postpartum.[5] Reabsorption of extravascular volume can also contribute to increased preload to the RV. CO continues to remain elevated for or up to 48 hours postdelivery. All these factors contribute to the development of acute RV failure.

Pulmonary Arterial Hypertension Outcomes in Pregnancy

Studies from the 1960s and 1970s first defined the extreme risk of pregnancy with PAH, reporting a maternal mortality of greater than 50%, with most deaths occurring in late gestation, during labor, or early in the postpartum period.[7,8] Data from a systematic overview of outcomes in 125 pregnant patients with PAH from 1978 through 1996 by Weiss and colleagues[6] defined an overall maternal mortality of 38%, with a range of 30% in idiopathic PAH, 36% in congenital disease/Eisenmenger syndrome, and 56% in secondary pulmonary hypertension (PH) (including PH associated with thromboembolic and connective tissue disease). A comparative analysis by Bedard and colleagues[8] of 73 pregnancies with PAH from 1997 to 2007 reported a significant decrease in overall maternal mortality (25% vs 38%; $P = .047$), with concomitant decreases in mortality within each cause of PH (17% in idiopathic PAH, 28% in congenital disease/Eisenmenger syndrome, and 33% in secondary PH). Most deaths occurred in the first month postpartum in both studies. Independent risk factors for maternal mortality were late diagnosis (odds ratio [OR] 5.4; $P = .002$), late presentation to the hospital (OR 1.1 per week of pregnancy; $P = .01$), primigravida (OR 3.70; $P = .03$) and the use of general anesthesia (OR 4.37; $P = .02$).[1,9]

Table 1 summarizes the results of key studies of maternal and fetal outcomes published to date with particular emphasis on improved maternal mortality outcomes and the more widespread utilization of PAH-specific therapies in the past 2 decades. The most recent report from a prospective, international registry by Jaïs and colleagues[10] followed 26 pregnant women with PAH and reported a significantly decreased maternal mortality (3 women died from right heart failure and 1 required urgent heart and lung transplantation); the investigators note that patients with successful

Table 1
Key studies of maternal and fetal outcomes in pregnancy with pulmonary arterial hypertension

Study	Total Number of Patients (n)	Pulmonary Arterial Hypertension Etiology (n)	Pulmonary Arterial Hypertension Therapy (n)	Overall Maternal Mortality (n)	Fetal Outcomes	Risk Factors for Maternal Mortality
Weiss et al,[6] (1978–1996)	n = 125	iPAH = 27 CHD = 73 APAH = 25	CCB = rare Digoxin = rare AC = 62	n = 48 (38%)	Died = 16	1. Late diagnosis (OR 5.4; P = .002) 2. Late presentation to hospital (OR 1.1 per week of pregnancy; P = .01)
Bonnin et al,[7] (1992–2002)	n = 14	iPAH = 4 CHD = 6 Other = 4	CCB = 1 Prostacyclin = 2 Digoxin = 2 AC = 2 iNO = 3	n = 5 (36%)	Stillbirth = 1 Aborted = 1 Died = 2	—
Bédard et al,[8] (1997–2007)	n = 73	iPAH = 29 CHD = 29 APAH = 15	None = 30 CCB = 19 PDE5-INH = 5 ERA = 2 Prostacyclin = 30 iNO = 19	n = 18 (25%)	Stillbirth = 1 Premature = 3	1. Primigravida (OR 3.70; P = .03) 2. General anesthesia (OR 4.37; P = .02).
Duarte et al,[9] (1999–2009)	n = 18	iPAH = 7 CHD = 8 Other = 3	None = 8 CCB = 1 PDE5-INH = 2 ERA = 8 Prostacyclin = 2	n = 5 (36%)	Stillbirth = 1 Aborted = 1 Died = 2	—
Kiely et al,[12] (2002–2009)	n = 10	iPAH = 3 CHD = 3 Other = 4	Prostacyclin = 8 PDE5-INH = 2	n = 1 (10%)	Aborted = 5	—
Katsuragi et al,[11] (1982–2007)	n = 42	iPAH = 7 CHD = 31 Other = 4	NR	n = 1 (2%)	Aborted = 18 Died = 1	Severe PAH: • PASP >50 mm Hg by TTE • mPAP >40 mm Hg by RHC
Jaïs et al,[10] (2007–2010)	n = 26	iPAH = 17 CHD = 1 Other = 8	None = 4 CCB = 8 PDE5-INH = 7 ERA = 7 Prostacyclin = 8 OAC = 13	n = 3 (12%)	Aborted = 8	High PVR: • Successful pregnancies: mean PVR = 500 ± 352 dyn·s·cm^{-5} • Maternal death: mean PVR = 1667 ± 209 dyn·s·cm^{-5}

Abbreviations: AC, anti-coagulation; APAH, associated pulmonary arterial hypertension; CHD, CHD-associated PAH/Eisenmenger syndrome; iPAH, idiopathic PAH; mpAP, mean pulmonary arterial pressure; NR, not reported; OAC, oral anticoagulants (warfarin); Other, other types of PH; PASP, PA systolic pressure; PDE5-INH, PDE5 inhibitors.

pregnancies had lower average PVR than those who died or required heart/lung transplantation (see **Table 1**). These results confirm the findings by Katsuragi and colleagues[11] reporting higher maternal mortality in patients with increasing severity of PAH defined as mean pulmonary arterial pressure greater than 40 mm Hg by right heart catheterization (RHC) (see **Table 1**).

Diagnosis of Pulmonary Arterial Hypertension in Pregnancy

Many symptoms of PAH, including dyspnea, lower extremity edema, weight gain, and dizziness, may be initially attributed to normal pregnancy. Plasma B-type natriuretic peptide remains a useful diagnostic tool with a high negative predictive value in pregnant patients with heart disease.[13] The authors recommend transthoracic echocardiography (TTE) as the best noninvasive screening method to estimate pulmonary artery (PA) pressures, evaluate right heart structure and function, and exclude competing left heart diagnoses, such as valvular disease or peripartum cardiomyopathy. Diagnosis should be confirmed by RHC via the internal jugular or brachial approach. There are minimal data to address specific complication rates associated with RHC in pregnant patients, although each patient should be counseled on the general risks of infection, thrombosis, pneumothorax, arrhythmias, and PA rupture.[14] A small study of 18 pregnant patients undergoing both TTE and RHC demonstrated that although there was good correlation between estimated RV systolic pressure by TTE and PA pressure by RHC (rho = 0.79; $P<.0001$), RHC eliminated the concern for PH in 30% of cases and should be performed when major decisions, such as pregnancy termination, rest on accurate diagnosis of PH.[15]

Management of Pulmonary Arterial Hypertension in Pregnancy

Despite advances in the treatment of PAH, which have brought some improvement in maternal mortality rates, the current guidelines continue to recommend contraception and avoidance of pregnancy; if a woman with PAH becomes pregnant despite extensive counseling and appropriate contraceptive measures, early termination of pregnancy should be discussed. If the patient declines termination, she should be referred to a PH center with a multidisciplinary team, including a PH specialist, high-risk obstetrician, and cardiac anesthesiologist early in pregnancy. Frequent monitoring with careful attention to functional status and RV assessment by echocardiography is essential especially late in the second and third trimesters. One referral center recommends monthly cardiology visits until 28 weeks gestation and weekly visits thereafter.[16] Medical and obstetric management of pregnancy in PAH is highly specialized and should abide by consideration of individual risks/benefits, but this article review the use of major classes of PAH agents in pregnancy. Pregnant patients were uniformly excluded from all clinical trials of PAH drugs and the evidence discussed comes from single-center case studies.

Clinicians caring for pregnant patients with PAH also should keep in mind that the physiologic changes of pregnancy, including increased plasma volume and accelerated hepatic metabolism and renal clearance, can alter the pharmacokinetics and plasma bioavailability of all these agents. Careful monitoring of drug effects and toxicities is required (**Table 2**).

Medical management

Calcium channel blockers The safety of calcium channel blockers (CCBs) in pregnancy has been well established outside of PAH, and CCBs have the additional advantage of reducing the incidence of preterm labor. Unfortunately, only 10% of PAH patients have a sustained response to CCB therapy.[17] The negative inotropic effects of CCBs limit their utility in acutely decompensated RV failure.

Phosphodiesterase-5 inhibitors Sildenafil causes dilatation of the pulmonary vasculature and, less so, the systemic circulation and may exert a positive inotropic effect on the RV. Several case series have reported sildenafil as generally well tolerated in pregnant patients and without teratogenic effects.[13,18,19] Tadalafil is a long-acting PDE5 inhibitor. To the authors' knowledge, there are no case reports of tadalafil use in pregnancy with PAH.

Endothelin receptor antagonists Bosentan, ambrisentan, and macitentan are known to be teratogenic (category X) and should be stopped as soon as pregnancy is suspected. The classification of ERAs as category X is based largely on data from reproductive studies of bosentan (Tracleer) in mice that demonstrated aortic arch malformations, ventricular septal defects, and craniofacial abnormalities in mice deficient in endothelin-1; further studies also showed that bosentan inhibits normal closure of the ductus arteriosus in rabbit and rat fetuses.[14,15]

Prostacyclin analogs Epoprostenol (Flolan and Veletri), an IV prostacyclin analog, is the only therapy shown to affect mortality in PAH and has been shown associated with favorable outcomes in several studies of pregnant women with severe

Table 2
US food and Drug Administration assigned pregnancy risk category for pulmonary arterial hypertension drugs

Drug	Pregnancy Risk Category
CCBs	
Diltiazem	C
Nifedipine	C
PDE5 inhibitors	
Sildenafil	B
Tadalafil	B
ERAs	
Bosentan	X
Ambrisentan	X
Macitentan	X
Prostacyclins	
Epoprostenol (IV)	B
Treprostinil (IV, subcutaneous)	B
Iloprost (inhaled)	C
Treprostinil (inhaled)	B
Soluble guanylate cyclase stimulator	
Riociguat	X
iNO	C

B: animal studies have failed to demonstrate a risk to the fetus and there are no adequate or well-controlled studies in pregnant women; C: Animal studies have shown an adverse effect on the fetus and there are no adequate and well-controlled studies in humans but potential benefits may warrant use of the drug in pregnant women despite potential risks; and X: studies in animals or humans have demonstrated fetal abnormalities or there is positive evidence of human fetal risk based on adverse reaction data from investigational or marketing experience, and the risks involved in use in pregnant women clearly outweigh the potential benefits.

PAH.[9,18,20,21] A small case series by Goland and colleagues describes 2 patients who presented with severe PAH in their third trimester. They were both treated with sildenafil and IV epoprostenol with successfully delivered healthy infants.[18] A key advantage of IV epoprostenol is a short half-life, which allows for rapid dose escalation. Prostacyclins inhibit platelet aggregation and may cause thrombocytopenia, so patients should be monitored for bleeding, especially during delivery and the immediate postpartum period. An experienced center recommends initiation of treatment with IV epoprostenol in all women with severe PAH and more than mild RV dilatation by 30 weeks gestation.[16] Patients should be continued on IV prostacyclins throughout delivery and well into the postpartum period after which consideration of weaning, replacement or augmentation with other PAH therapies are dependent on severity of PAH and clinical status of the patient.

Iloprost (Ventavis) is a synthetic inhaled prostacyclin analog similar to epoprostenol in its mechanism of action. IV administration of iloprost has been shown to increase the risk of shortened digits in rat pups at doses of 0.01 mg/kg/d but did not demonstrate similar teratogenic effects in rabbits or monkeys even at doses up to 40 mg/kd/d.[22] A small study of 3 women with diverse etiologies of PAH treated with inhaled iloprost starting as early as 8 weeks' gestation resulted in uncomplicated deliveries with no congenital abnormalities in the infants.[23]

Soluble guanylate cyclase stimulator Riociguat (Adempas), a soluble guanylate cyclase stimulator, is a novel therapeutic agent shown to improve exercise tolerance, pulmonary hemodynamics, and World Health Organization functional class in PAH[24] as well as PH due to inoperable chronic thromboembolic disease.[25] Riociguat demonstrated significant teratogenicity in preclinical studies and is strictly contraindicated in pregnancy (category X).[26] Riociguat prescriptions to women are available only through a restricted program called the Adempas Risk Evaluation and Mitigation Strategies program.

Inhaled nitric oxide Inhaled nitric oxide (iNO) is a potent and direct pulmonary vasodilator often used as a rescue medication in critically ill pregnant patients with PAH and acute RV failure. iNO must be slowly weaned due to the risk of rebound PH after sudden discontinuation. Long-term use carries additional risks of methemoglobinemia.

Anticoagulation The practice of anticoagulation in patients with PAH is not standardized due to the paucity of data, although most clinicians agree that thromboprophylaxis should be considered in women with PAH during pregnancy and in the postpartum period, if no significant contraindications are present.[7,8,12] Full-dose anticoagulation should be continued when other indications, such as thromboembolism and atrial fibrillation, exist. In the systematic review by Bédard and colleagues,[8] 52% of patients with PAH and 24% of congenital heart disease (CHD)–associated PAH were treated with anticoagulation during pregnancy. Older studies suggested that anticoagulation may be harmful in patients with Eisenmenger syndrome who are prone to excessive bleeding[27]; however, women with Eisenmenger syndrome and a patent foramen ovale are at higher risk for paradoxic emboli so may have a stronger indication for prophylactic anticoagulation.[2] Heparin and low-molecular-weight heparin are most commonly used because they do not cross the placenta, whereas warfarin does cross the placental barrier and can cause fetal defects, including nasal hypoplasia and stippled epiphyses.[2] The novel oral anticoagulants should be avoided in pregnant women with PAH given the paucity of data associated with their use.

Mode of delivery

The timing and mode of delivery should be carefully planned in advance with consideration of scheduled early delivery at fetal maturity (32–36 weeks). Both vaginal delivery and caesarean section present distinct risks to the pregnant patient with PAH: vaginal delivery is associated with a larger risk of rapid changes to venous return/preload with repeated Valsalva maneuvers during the second stage of labor and due to vasovagal reactions to pain but carries an overall lower risk of hemorrhage, thromboembolism, and infection compared with caesarean section.[6] Several experts in the field still strongly advocate for scheduled caesarean section as the preferred mode of delivery.[3,7,12]

If vaginal delivery is chosen, the left lateral decubitus position should be used to decrease the risk of compression of the inferior vena cava by the uterus. Prolonged second stage of labor should be strictly avoided and assisted delivery with forceps or vacuum considered in all patients with PAH. Uterotonic agents, such as ergometrine and carboprost, should not be used because they can cause pulmonary vasoconstriction and bronchospasm, leading to cardiovascular collapse.[16] Furthermore, in 1 case report, oxytocin use in 2 pregnant patients with advanced PAH was shown to cause increased PVR and acute RV failure.[28]

Epidural or combined spinal-epidural anesthesia should be performed by an experienced anesthesiologist. Gradual dosing of epidural anesthesia is mandatory to minimize the risk of systemic hypotension. Studies have reported that combined low-dose spinal-epidural anesthesia provides better sensory block with fewer blood pressure–lowering effects.[7,19] Regardless of the anesthetic management strategy, effective analgesia is essential to avoid vasovagal reactions and pain-related tachycardia.

Peripartum and postpartum management

Most patients with PAH require close hemodynamic monitoring with telemetry and frequent vital sign assessment at the onset of labor. ICU level of care with central venous and arterial lines may be necessary in the peripartum period. The use of a Swan-Ganz catheter is controversial because it exposes patients to the risks of infection, thrombotic events, and PA rupture but may be considered in a select group of very high-risk patients, if it informs management decisions.[8]

The risks of rapid hemodynamic fluctuations remain high in the immediate postpartum period. Patients should be observed in the ICU for several days after delivery.

Summary

Despite an improvement in maternal outcomes with the advent of modern PAH therapies and multidisciplinary delivery management strategies, pregnancy remains a high-risk hemodynamic state in PAH and should be avoided. Reported risk factors for maternal mortality include late presentation, primigravida status, and general anesthesia. Newer studies show that patients with well-controlled PAH (lower pulmonary pressures and PVR) have better outcomes. If pregnancy occurs, management should include a multidisciplinary team of PAH specialists, high-risk obstetricians, and cardiac anesthesiologists. PAH therapies, including CCBs, PDE5 inhibitors, and prostacyclins, should generally be continued through delivery, whereas ERAs and riociguat are category X and should be discontinued. IV and inhaled prostacyclins can be initiated during pregnancy to stabilize hemodynamics. Therapeutic anticoagulation should be maintained during pregnancy, although heparin and low-molecular-weight heparin are favored over warfarin. In patients not on therapeutic anticoagulation prepregnancy, thromboprophylaxis should be initiated. Delivery mode should be individualized for each patient by the multidisciplinary team and planned for 34 weeks gestation if possible. Combined low-dose spinal-epidural anesthesia may be the preferred approach, with careful attention to avoidance of large volume shifts, systemic hypotension, hypoxemia, tachycardia, and acidosis. Individualized counseling of the expectant mother about the risks of pregnancy, effective contraception, and potential teratogenicity of PAH drugs is paramount.

RIGHT VENTRICULAR FAILURE
Introduction

Progressive RV failure remains the most common cause of death in patients with PAH, and RV systolic function is the most important determinant of prognosis in PAH.[29–31] RV failure is characterized by an elevated RV filling pressure (right atrial pressure [RAP] >8 mm Hg) and a low cardiac index (cardiac index <2.5 L/min/m²). This article reviews the pathophysiology of RV failure due to PAH, the diagnostic features of RV failure, and the management of RV failure with emphasis on the acutely decompensated phase.

Anatomy and Physiology of the Right Ventricle

The RV has a distinct embryologic origin and differs in its anatomy and physiology from the left ventricle (LV). The RV has a tripartite structure with an inlet (sinus), chamber, and outlet (conus). Distinguishing anatomic features include heavy trabeculae, a moderator band, and absence of fibrous continuity between the inlet and outlet valves. Unlike the ellipsoid LV, the RV has a complex geometry and appears triangular in the longitudinal plane and crescent-shaped in the short-axis plane. The RV myocardium comprises transverse and longitudinal fibers rather than the circumferentially oriented myocyte networks of the LV, and longitudinal shortening contributes more to RV SV than circumferential shortening.[32,33] The RV contracts sequentially from inflow to outflow with most contraction occurring along the longitudinal axis. The RV is a thin-walled structure that contains approximately one-sixth of the muscle mass of the LV but generates the same SV at a fraction of the stroke work because of the low resistance and high capacitance of the normal pulmonary vasculature.

Pathophysiology of Right Ventricular Failure in Pulmonary Arterial Hypertension

The pathophysiology of RV failure in PAH is summarized in **Fig. 1**.

The RV is a low-pressure, high-compliance chamber poorly designed to handle chronic elevation in afterload associated with PAH. In the early stages, there is a compensated phase with adaptive, concentric RV hypertrophy in response to increased wall stress; this phase is characterized by a normal RAP and normal CO, and patients typically experience few symptoms. In the declining phase, there is maladaptive RV hypertrophy and interstitial fibrosis as well as increasing diastolic dysfunction. Rising RAP is required to maintain an adequate CO, and patients become symptomatic with exercise. The RV dilates, resulting in increased wall stress and increased RV myocardial consumption, which leads to RV ischemia and progressive systolic/diastolic failure, which is the hallmark of the final decompensated phase. Progressive RV dilatation ultimately leads to right-to-left shift of the interventricular septum during diastole, which compromises LV diastolic filling and leads to decreased LV preload and low systemic CO. The decompensated phase is characterized by high RAP, low CO, and symptoms with minimal activity or at rest.[24]

Diagnosis of Right Ventricular Failure

Physical examination

The symptoms of RV failure include severe dyspnea, chest pain, fatigue, and presyncope/syncope. On physical examination, a loud P2 sound due to accentuated pulmonic valve closure is present in more than 90% of patients. Other symptoms include jugular venous distention, peripheral edema, right-sided S3 gallop, RV lift, enlarged/pulsatile liver, and ascites. A low systemic blood pressure with a narrow pulse pressure and cool extremities are evidence of peripheral tissue and vital organ hypoperfusion and resultant peripheral vasoconstriction.[25,26,34]

Transthoracic echocardiography

TTE remains the first-line imaging modality to evaluate RV function. The RV typically appears dilated and hypertrophied with reduced systolic function assessed by the fractional area change and tricuspid annular plane systolic excursion. Pulsed-wave Doppler in the RV outflow tract typically reveals a reduced velocity time integral, suggesting low CO; in addition, midsystolic deceleration, or notching, of the RV outflow tract velocity time integral is especially suggestive of high PVR.[35] In the parasternal short-axis view, the LV appears crescent-shaped, or D-shaped, as the interventricular septum flattens toward the LV. Septal flattening during systole suggests RV pressure overload, whereas septal flattening during diastole suggests RV volume overload; in cases of RV failure, septal flattening is usually seen throughout the cardiac cycle.[24]

Pulmonary vascular capacitance, defined as the ratio of the SV (mL) divided by the PA pulse pressure (mm Hg), has been shown to be a strong predictor of survival in PAH (hazard ratio 17.0 per mL/mm Hg decrease; 95% CI, 13.0–22.0; $P<.0001$), outperforming all other RHC parameters.[36] Doppler echocardiography can reliably estimate pulmonary vascular capacitance noninvasively according to the equation, $SV/4(TR^2-PR^2)$, and was a more powerful predictor of survival than conventional echocardiographic and invasive hemodynamic measurements in a cohort of 54 PAH patients.[37] Capacitance, or compliance, takes into account the oscillatory load due to pulsatile blood flow so it is equally important to calculate as the PVR, which assumes a static load (mean pressure/mean flow). A study by Lankhaar and colleagues[38] demonstrated that both resistance (R) and compliance (C) change with PH therapy whereas their product (RC) remains

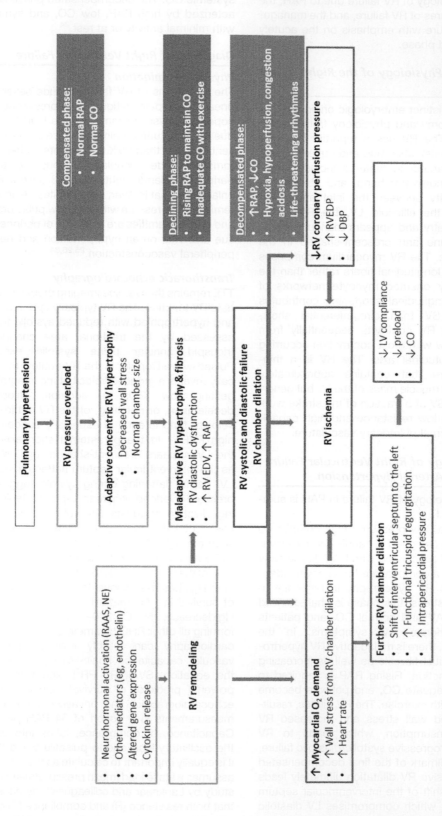

Fig. 1. Pathophysiology of RV failure in PAH. DBP, diastolic blood pressure; EDV, end diastolic volume; NE, norepinephrine; RAP, right atrial pressure; RAAS, renin-angiotensin-aldosterone system; RVEDP, RV end-diastolic pressure. (*Data from* DeMarco T. Managing right ventricular failure in PAH: an algorithmic approach. Adv PH 2005;4(4):16–26; with permission.)

constant, suggesting that R and C are inversely coupled; in addition, changes in both R and C predicted changes in cardiac index with PH therapy.

Hemodynamic monitoring

The use of PA catheters has been questioned in distributive and cardiogenic shock,[39,40] and its use in the management of acute RV failure is likewise controversial.[41] PA catheter placement enables measurement of RAP, PA wedge pressure, CO, and mixed venous oxygen saturation (Mvo$_2$). In PAH, the PA wedge pressure is low and real-time measurement of PVR is not always useful; in addition, insertion of the PA catheter may be challenging in patients with PAH.[41] The authors favor using a central line to monitor central venous pressure and superior vena cava oxygen saturation to guide treatment in addition to other markers of tissue perfusion, such as renal and liver function tests, urine output, and lactate levels. The use of superior vena cava oxygen saturation to predict PA oxygen saturation (Mvo$_2$) has been well validated in a cohort of patients with PAH receiving IV prostanoid therapy (r = 0.91; P<.001).[42]

Management of Right Ventricular Failure in Pulmonary Arterial Hyptension

Chronic right ventricular failure management

Medical therapy The long-term management of RV failure requires aggressive management of PAH with evidence-based therapies, as discussed elsewhere in this issue (see Barnett CF, Alvarez P, Park MH: Pulmonary Arterial Hypertension: Diagnosis and Treatment, in this issue). Lowering RV afterload and reducing wall stress with PA vasodilators (oxygen, PDE5 inhibitors, ERAs, and prostacyclin analogs) is a key strategy to prevent RV failure.[41] Diuretic therapy to maintain euvolemia offers another opportunity to reduce RV wall stress by decreased preload and degree of tricuspid regurgitation. Although loop diuretics are the mainstay of therapy, their effects can be augmented with potent thiazide diuretic antagonists in cases of diuretic resistance. Aldosterone antagonists block the deleterious effects of aldosterone activation, including sodium/fluid retention, increase in RV mass/fibrosis, and endothelial dysfunction, and should be a mainstay of therapy for chronic RV failure.[41] β-Blockers and CCBs should be avoided when CO is reduced. Although controversial, low-dose digoxin (0.125 mg daily) may be useful adjunctive therapy in chronic RV failure because it has been shown to have positive RV inotropic effects (increasing the CO by approximately 10%) and to decrease levels of circulating catecholamines.[43]

Atrial septostomy Percutaneous balloon atrial septostomy (BAS) creates a perforation in the atrial septum and allows right-to-left shunting of blood to reduce high right-sided filling pressures and improve LV filling. BAS is indicated for severe PAH with recurrent syncope and has been used for RV failure refractory to maximal medical management or as a bridge to lung transplantation. BAS should be performed in hemodynamically stable patients without significant hypoxemia because the risk of fatal complications is high in those with RAP greater than 20 mm Hg and oxygen saturation measured by pulse oximetry less than 80% on room air.[44]

Mechanical circulatory support ECMO has been reported as an effective treatment strategy in patients with PH and massive PE. ECMO can be rapidly implanted (typically via femoral venous and arterial cannulation) but risks include vessel injury, thromboembolism, bleeding, and infection.[45] At least 1 case series describes 5 patients with severe RV failure and progressive organ dysfunction treated with prolonged ECMO support (18–35 days) and successfully bridged to lung transplantation in 4 of 5 cases.[46] The interventional lung assist device, NovaLung iLA (NovaLung, Hechingen, Germany), is a pumpless, low-resistance diffusion membrane rescue device used as a bridge to lung transplantation in patients with ventilation-refractory hypoxia since 2003.[47] When implanted as a PA to left atrium (PA-LA) bypass, it creates a right-to-left shunt that unloads the RV and improves LV filling.[48] Although PA-LA NovaLung requires central cannulation via a sternotomy, it allows for patient mobilization and can be used as a long-term bridge, with reported duration of support up to 174 days in an experienced center in Toronto.[48] Other case reports of successful bridge to transplant with PA-LA NovaLung have been published.[49]

Right-sided ventricular assist devices have been used to provide RV support after orthotopic heart transplantation or left-sided ventricular assist device implantation but have not been used to treat PAH-associated RV failure due to risks of pulmonary microcirculatory hemorrhage associated with the introduction of a high-flow pump into a diseased vasculature.[50] There are 2 devices currently approved by the US Food and Drug Administration for RV support: Thoratec PVAD for long-term support and CentriMag for short-term support (both by Thoratec, Pleasanton, California). Permanent support, or destination therapy, has not been investigated.

Lung and heart-lung transplantation Bilateral lung transplantation is an established therapeutic option for advanced PAH with refractory RV failure, with reported survival rates of 70% at 1 year.[51] Long-term survival is in large part determined by the development of post-transplant bronchiolitis obliterans.[24] Heart-lung transplantation has been performed for complex CHD with PAH. Indications for heart-lung transplantation include irreversible myocardial dysfunction or congenital defects with irreparable defects of the values or chambers in conjunction with intrinsic lung disease or severe PAH. The timing of transplantation can be challenging; however, patients commonly have sequela of RV failure, such as persistent World Health Organization functional class IV systems on maximal medical therapy, reduced cardiac index less than 2.0 L/min/m², and RAP greater than 15 mm Hg.[52]

Acute right ventricular failure management
Management of RV failure rests on the principles of decreasing preload, improving contractility, and reducing afterload, with the goals of optimizing systemic perfusion and oxygenation (**Fig. 2**). There are no controlled clinical trials addressing the treatment of acute decompensated RV failure, and the following management strategies are based on key review articles by experts in the field and the authors' experience.

Correction of triggering factors Triggering factors, such as dietary or medication noncompliance, arrhythmias, infection, and pregnancy, can be identified in many cases of acutely decompensated RV failure. Timely identification of these triggers is key to successful treatment. A single-center prospective study of 46 patients with PAH admitted to the ICU for RV failure identified triggering factor in 41% (n = 19) of the admissions; these included unplanned withdrawal of therapy (n = 4), infection (n = 10), and arrhythmias (n = 3).[53] The same study highlights the very high mortality associated with RV failure requiring ICU admission: 41.3% (n = 19) of patients died in the ICU and an additional 13% (n = 6) died within 3 months of hospital discharge. Serum B-type natriuretic peptide, C-reactive protein, sodium, and creatinine on admission correlated with survival but documented infection was the single strongest predictor of death (74% of non-survivors vs 22% of survivors; $P = .0005$).[53] Patients with chronic PAH are at risk for both Gram-positive and Gram-negative septicemia due to frequent presence of indwelling central venous catheters[24] and the loss of gut barrier function as the result of venous congestion and

low CO.[54] Atrial tachyarrhythmias should be aggressively managed with emphasis on rhythm control rather than rate control, because atrial contractility makes a crucial contribution to CO in RV failure.[54] β-Blockers and CCBs should generally be avoided because of their negative inotropic effects. Digoxin, amiodarone, electrical cardioversion, and radiofrequency ablation (for atrial flutter or refractory atrial fibrillation) have been used successfully in our center.

Restoration of oxygenation Correction of hypoxemia with supplemental oxygen to an arterial oxygen saturation greater than 90% is critical because pulmonary vessels constrict with hypoxia (Euler-Liljestrand reflex) and relax with hyperoxia.[55] Correction of significant anemia and iron deficiency helps improve delivery of oxygen to hypoxic tissues; some investigators have recommended a goal hemoglobin of 10 g/dL in the setting of RV failure.[54]

Endotracheal intubation and mechanical ventilation are fraught with danger in the setting of RV failure. Several case reports have reported cardio-circulatory collapse after anesthesia induction and initiation of positive-pressure ventilation (PPV).[56,57] Sedatives decrease sympathetic tone and SVR whereas PPV impedes systemic venous return, which causes a dramatic lowering of LV filling pressures and allows for more profound right-to-left shifting of the interventricular septum. At the same time, PPV-mediated increases in PVR lead to acute RV pressure overload with RV dilatation and decrease in RV systolic function causing an even more pronounced leftward shift of the interventricular septum.[57,58] High positive end-expiratory pressure (PEEP) can increase the RV end-diastolic pressure leading to a reduction in RV coronary perfusion pressure and RV ischemia; at the same time, high PEEP can lead to decreased RV filling and SV.[43] Studies of postoperative patients suggest that PEEP greater than 15 cm H_2O is sufficient to cause an increase in RV volume and a decrease in RV ejection fraction.[59]

If mechanical ventilation cannot be avoided, etomidate is the preferred induction agent.[60] Systemic hypotension should be treated aggressively. The lowest possible PEEP settings should be used while avoiding hypercapnia, academia, and alveolar hypoxia.

Maintenance of cardiac output and systemic perfusion Initiation or augmentation of pulmonary vasodilators allows for stabilization of CO and systemic blood pressure. IV prostacyclin derivatives (epoprostenol, treprosinil, and iloprost) are the initial treatment of choice, and the authors favor

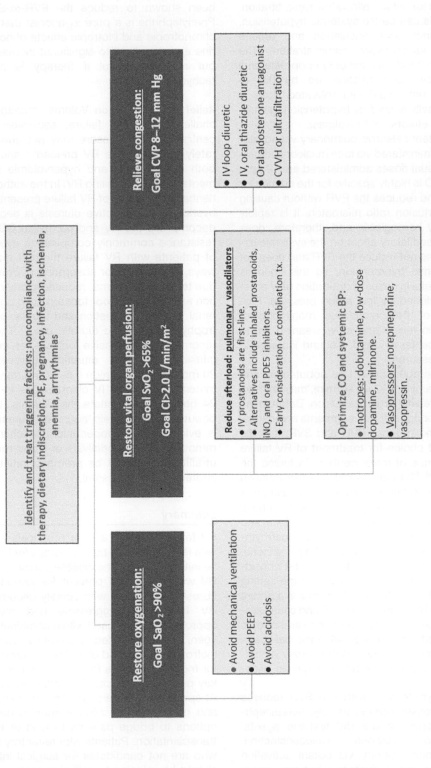

Fig. 2. Hemodynamic management of patients with acute RV failure. Svo₂ Mixed venous oxygen saturation. BP, blood pressure; CVP, central venous pressure; CVVH, continuous veno-venous hemofiltration; PE, pulmonary embolism; SaO2, arterial oxygen saturation; SvO2, venous oxygen saturation.

IV epoprostenol (Flolan and Veletri) because of the demonstrated mortality benefit in randomized controlled trials of PAH as well as its short half-life (3–5 minutes), which allows for rapid titration. All prostanoids can cause systemic hypotension, which can limit dose escalation and require concomitant vasopressor administration. The authors recommend initiation of IV epoprosterenol at 1 ng/kg/min and titrating up by 0.5 to 1 mg/kg/min until maximum tolerated dose is reached (typically limited by hypotension, gastrointestinal side effects, and myalgias).

iNO is a potent selective pulmonary vasodilator that can be administered via face mask or endotracheal tube. Usual doses administered are 10 ppm to 20 ppm. iNO is highly specific for the pulmonary vasculature and reduces the PVR without causing ventilation perfusion ratio mismatch. It is rapidly inactivated by hemoglobin and, therefore, does not exert a vasodilatory effect on the systemic circulation. It does not reduce the SVR and does not lead to systemic hypotension, so this agent is particularly useful in cases of uptitration of IV prostacyclins precluded by low blood pressure. Prolonged use of iNO mandates monitoring of methemoglobin levels and slow weaning (in 1–5 ppm increments) to avoid rebound increase in pulmonary pressures.

β-Adrenergic agents, such as dobutamine and low-dose dopamine (1–2 μg/kg/min), may improve CO and restore vital organ perfusion. Dobutamine is a $β_1$-receptor agonist that augments myocardial contractility and reduces PVR and SVR; it is the initial agent of choice for treatment of RV failure in the experience of many centers, including the authors'.[41,53,61] The authors recommend initiation of dobutamine at 2 μg/kg/min and increasing to a maximum of 5 μg/kg/min guided by mixed venous oxygen saturation levels. Both dobutamine and dopamine carry the risk of atrial tachycarrhythmias; if these become therapy limiting, milrinone, a PDE3 inhibitor and inodilator, may be considered. Milrinone may also be useful in the setting of chronic β-blocker therapy. Milrinone is a potent vasodilator and may decrease SVR and cause systemic hypotension out of proportion to its inotropic effects. Inhaled aerosolized milrinone has been shown to cause more selective pulmonary vasodilation in case reports but has not gained widespread use.[62]

Systemic hypotension with low SVR requires use of vasopressor agents: usually, norepinephrine and vasopressin are the first-line agents. Norepinephrine provides vasoconstriction, chronotropy, and inotropy via potent activation of $α_1$-receptors and $β_1$-receptors but may cause pulmonary vasoconstriction and tachycardia at high doses.[45] Vasopressin causes systemic vasoconstriction via the V1 receptor but may actually cause pulmonary vasodilation at low dose. It has been shown to reduce the PVR-to-SVR ratio. Phenylephrine is a pure $α_1$-agonist that lacks the chronotropic and inotropic effects of norepinephrine and may lead to significant increase in PVR but may be useful if therapy is limited by tachycardia.[45]

Relief of congestion Volume management is challenging in RV failure, especially because central venous pressure may not always accurately estimate true RV preload[63] and because both hypovolemia and hypervolemia are detrimental to CO in a failing RV. In the authors' experience, most cases of RV failure present with fluid overload, and effective diuresis is necessary to decompress the RV and normalize CO. Diuretic resistance commonly complicates management of patients with RV failure through many pathways, including poor absorption of oral diuretics due to gut wall edema, reduced glomerular filtration as a result of poor forward flow, and passive renal venous congestion and tubular cell hypertrophy from chronic diuretic use.[41] The authors recommend aggressive boluses or continuous infusion of loop diuretics (furosemide 5–20 mg/h or bumetanide 0.5–2.0 mg/h) with intermittent addition of IV chlorthiazide (1–2 g over 24 hours) to potentiate the diuresis. Low-dose dobutamine may help augment diuresis if there is evidence of hypoperfusion. Mechanical fluid removal with hemodialysis or other methods of utrafiltration should be promptly initiated if this strategy is unsuccessful.

Summary

RV failure predicts a poor prognosis in patients with PAH. Evidence-based therapy for PAH should be initiated early in the disease course to decrease RV wall stress and prevent RV remodeling and fibrosis. In patients with acutely decompensated RV failure, an aggressive and multifaceted approach must be used with a combination of oxygen, IV or inhaled pulmonary vasodilators, inotropic agents, and diuretics; a thorough search for triggering factors for the decompensation is a key part of the successful management strategy. At specialized centers, atrial septostomy, ECMO, and mechanical circulatory support devices are options to bridge patients to lung or heart-lung transplantation. Patients with refractory RV failure who are not candidates for surgical intervention should be referred to palliative care to maximize quality of life and symptom relief.

REFERENCES

1. Pitkin RM, Perloff JK, Koos BJ, et al. Pregnancy and congenital heart disease. Ann Intern Med 1990; 112(6):445–54.

2. Običan SG, Cleary KL. Pulmonary arterial hypertension in pregnancy. Semin Perinatol 2015;38(5): 289–94.

3. Safdar Z. Pulmonary arterial hypertension in pregnant women. Ther Adv Respir Dis 2013;7(1):51–63.

4. Marik PE, Plante LA. Venous thromboembolic disease and pregnancy. N Engl J Med 2008;359(19): 2025–33.

5. Stone SE, Morris TA. Pulmonary embolism during and after pregnancy. Crit Care Med 2005;33(Suppl 10):S294–300.

6. Weiss BM, Zemp L, Seifert B, et al. Outcome of pulmonary vascular disease in pregnancy: a systematic overview from 1978 through 1996. J Am Coll Cardiol 1998;31(7):1650–7.

7. Bonnin M, Mercier FJ, Sitbon O, et al. Severe pulmonary hypertension during pregnancy: mode of delivery and anesthetic management of 15 consecutive cases. Anesthesiology 2005;102(6):1133–7 [discussion: 5A–6A].

8. Bédard E, Dimopoulos K, Gatzoulis MA. Has there been any progress made on pregnancy outcomes among women with pulmonary arterial hypertension? Eur Heart J 2009;30(3):256–65.

9. Duarte AG, Thomas S, Safdar Z, et al. Management of pulmonary arterial hypertension during pregnancy: a retrospective, multicenter experience. Chest 2013;143(5):1330–6.

10. Jaïs X, Olsson KM, Barbera JA, et al. Pregnancy outcomes in pulmonary arterial hypertension in the modern management era. Eur Respir J 2012;40(4): 881–5. Available at: http://erj.ersjournals.com/ content/40/4/881.abstract.

11. Katsuragi S, Yamanaka K, Neki R, et al. Maternal outcome in pregnancy complicated with pulmonary arterial hypertension. Circ J 2012;76(9):2249–54.

12. Kiely DG, Condliffe R, Webster V, et al. Improved survival in pregnancy and pulmonary hypertension using a multiprofessional approach. BJOG 2010; 117(5):565–74.

13. Taçoy G, Ekim NN, Çengel A. Dramatic response of a patient with pregnancy induced idiopathic pulmonary arterial hypertension to sildenafil treatment. J Obstet Gynaecol Res 2010;36(2):414–7.

14. Kurihara Y, Kurihara H, Oda H, et al. Aortic arch malformations and ventricular septal defect in mice deficient in endothelin-1. J Clin Invest 1995; 96(1):293–300.

15. Shen J, Nakanishi T, Gu H, et al. The role of endothelin in oxygen-induced contraction of the ductus arteriosus in rabbit and rat fetuses. Heart Vessels 2002; 16(5):181–8.

16. Tabarsi N, Levy R, Rychel V, et al. Pregnancy among women with pulmonary arterial hypertension: a changing landscape? Int J Cardiol 2015;177(2):490–1.

17. Humbert M, Sitbon O, Simonneau G. Treatment of pulmonary arterial hypertension. N Engl J Med 2004;351(14):1425–36.

18. Goland S, Tsai F, Habib M, et al. Favorable outcome of pregnancy with an elective Use of epoprostenol and sildenafil in women with severe pulmonary hypertension. Cardiology 2010;115(3): 205–8. Available at: http://www.karger.com/DOI/ 10.1159/000287638.

19. Hsu C-H, Gomberg-Maitland M, Glassner C, et al. The management of pregnancy and pregnancy-related medical conditions in pulmonary arterial hypertension patients. Int J Clin Pract Suppl 2011; 172:6–14.

20. Badalian SS, Silverman RK, Aubry RH, et al. Twin pregnancy in a woman on long-term epoprostenol therapy for primary pulmonary hypertension. A case report. J Reprod Med 2000;45(2):149–52.

21. Zwicke DL, Buggy BP. Pregnancy and pulmonary arterial hypertension: successful management of 37 consecutive patients. Chest 2008;134(4_Meeting Abstracts):s64002. Available at: http://dx.doi.org/10. 1378/chest.134.4_MeetingAbstracts.s64002.

22. Battenfeld R, Schuh W, Schobel C. Studies on reproductive toxicity of iloprost in rats, rabbits and monkeys. Toxicol Lett 1995;78(3):223–34.

23. Elliot CA, Stewart P, Webster VJ, et al. The use of iloprost in early pregnancy in patients with pulmonary arterial hypertension. Eur Respir J 2005; 26(1):168–73.

24. DeMarco T. Managing right ventricular failure in PAH: an algorithmic approach. Advances in Pulmonary Hypertension 2005;4(4):16–26. Available at: http://www.phaonlineuniv.org/Journal/Article.cfm? ItemNumber=650. Accessed April 6, 2016.

25. McLaughlin VV, Archer SL, Badesch DB, et al. ACCF/AHA 2009 expert consensus document on pulmonary hypertension a report of the American College of cardiology Foundation Task Force on expert consensus Documents and the American heart association developed in collaboration with the American College of chest Physicians; American Thoracic Society, Inc.; and the pulmonary hypertension association. J Am Coll Cardiol 2009;53(17): 1573–619.

26. Rich S, Dantzker DR, Ayres SM, et al. Primary pulmonary hypertension. A national prospective study. Ann Intern Med 1987;107(2):216–23.

27. Pitts JA, Crosby WM, Basta LL. Eisenmenger's syndrome in pregnancy: does heparin prophylaxis improve the maternal mortality rate? Am Heart J 1977;93(3):321–6.

28. Price LC, Forrest P, Sodhi V, et al. Use of vasopressin after Caesarean section in idiopathic

pulmonary arterial hypertension. Br J Anaesth 2007; 99(4):552–5.

29. Chin KM, Kim NHS, Rubin LJ. The right ventricle in pulmonary hypertension. Coron Artery Dis 2005; 16(1):13–8.

30. Sandoval J, Bauerle O, Palomar A, et al. Survival in primary pulmonary hypertension. Validation of a prognostic equation. Circulation 1994;89(4): 1733–44.

31. D'Alonzo GE, Barst RJ, Ayres SM, et al. Survival in patients with primary pulmonary hypertension. Results from a national prospective registry. Ann Intern Med 1991;115(5):343–9.

32. Smerup M, Nielsen E, Agger P, et al. The three-dimensional arrangement of the myocytes aggregated together within the mammalian ventricular myocardium. Anat Rec (Hoboken) 2009;292(1): 1–11.

33. Voelkel NF, Quaife RA, Leinwand LA, et al. Right ventricular function and failure: report of a National Heart, Lung, and Blood Institute working group on cellular and molecular mechanisms of right heart failure. Circulation 2006;114(17):1883–91.

34. McGoon M, Gutterman D, Steen V, et al. Screening, early detection, and diagnosis of pulmonary arterial hypertension: ACCP evidence-based clinical practice guidelines. Chest 2004;126(Suppl 1):14S–34S.

35. Arkles JS, Opotowsky AR, Ojeda J, et al. Shape of the right ventricular doppler Envelope predicts hemodynamics and right heart function in pulmonary hypertension. Am J Respir Crit Care Med 2011; 183:268–76.

36. Mahapatra S, Nishimura RA, Sorajja P, et al. Relationship of pulmonary arterial capacitance and mortality in idiopathic pulmonary arterial hypertension. J Am Coll Cardiol 2006;47(4):799–803.

37. Mahapatra S, Nishimura R a, Oh JK, et al. The prognostic value of pulmonary vascular capacitance determined by doppler echocardiography in patients with pulmonary arterial hypertension. J Am Soc Echocardiogr 2006;19(8):1045–50.

38. Lankhaar J-W, Westerhof N, Faes TJC, et al. Pulmonary vascular resistance and compliance stay inversely related during treatment of pulmonary hypertension. Eur Heart J 2008;29(13):1688–95.

39. Harvey S, Harrison DA, Singer M, et al. Assessment of the clinical effectiveness of pulmonary artery catheters in management of patients in intensive care (PAC-Man): a randomised controlled trial. Lancet 2005;366(9484):472–7.

40. Sandham JD, Hull RD, Brant RF, et al. A randomized, controlled trial of the use of pulmonary-artery catheters in high-risk surgical patients. N Engl J Med 2003;348(1):5–14.

41. Sood N. Managing an acutely ill patient with pulmonary arterial hypertension. Expert Rev Respir Med 2013;7(1):77–83.

42. Chin KM. Central venous blood oxygen saturation monitoring in patients with chronic pulmonary arterial hypertension treated with continuous IV epoprostenol: correlation with measurements of hemodynamics and plasma brain natriuretic peptide levels. Chest 2007;132(3):786.

43. Buckley D, Gillham M. Invasive Respiratory Support. In: Sidebotham D, Mckee A, Gillham M, et al, editors. Cardiothorac Crit Care. Philadelphia: Elsevier; 2007. p. 419–36.

44. Galie N, Hoeper MM, Humbert M, et al. Guidelines for the diagnosis and treatment of pulmonary hypertension. Eur Respir J 2009;34(6):1219–63.

45. Price LC, Wort SJ, Finney SJ, et al. Pulmonary vascular and right ventricular dysfunction in adult critical care: current and emerging options for management: a systematic literature review. Crit Care 2010;14(5):R169.

46. Olsson, Karen M, Simon A, et al. Extracorporeal membrane oxygenation in nonintubated patients as bridge to lung transplantation. Am J Transplant 2010;10:2173–8.

47. Fischer S, Simon AR, Welte T, et al. Bridge to lung transplantation with the novel pumpless interventional lung assist device NovaLung. J Thorac Cardiovasc Surg 2006;131(3):719–23.

48. Granton J, Mercier O, De Perrot M. Management of severe pulmonary arterial hypertension. Semin Respir Crit Care Med 2013;34(5):700–13.

49. Patil NP, Mohite PN, Reed A, et al. Modified technique using Novalung as bridge to transplant in pulmonary hypertension. Ann Thorac Surg 2015;99(2):719–21.

50. Gomez-Arroyo J, Sandoval J, Simon MA, et al. Treatment for pulmonary arterial hypertesion-associated right ventricular dysfunction. Ann Am Thorac Soc 2014;11(7):1101–15.

51. Mendeloff EN, Meyers BF, Sundt TM, et al. Lung transplantation in pulmonary vascular disease. Ann Thorac Surg 2002;73:209–17.

52. Weill D, Benden C, Corris PA, et al. A consensus document for the selection of lung transplant candidates: 2014–an update from the pulmonary transplantation council of the international society for heart and lung transplantation. J Heart Lung Transplant 2015;34(1):1–15.

53. Sztrymf B, Souza R, Bertoletti L, et al. Prognostic factors of acute heart failure in patients with pulmonary arterial hypertension. Eur Respir J 2010;35(6): 1286–93.

54. Hoeper MM, Granton J. Intensive care unit management of patients with severe pulmonary hypertension and right heart failure. Am J Respir Crit Care Med 2011;184(10):1114–24.

55. Fischer LG, Van Aken H, Bürkle H. Management of pulmonary hypertension: physiological and pharmacological considerations for anesthesiologists. Anesth Analg 2003;96(6):1603–16.

56. Myles PS, Hall JL, Berry CB, et al. Primary pulmonary hypertension: prolonged cardiac arrest and successful resuscitation following induction of anesthesia for heart-lung transplantation. J Cardiothorac Vasc Anesth 1994;8(6):678–81.

57. Hohn L, Schweizer A, Morel DR, et al. Circulatory failure after anesthesia induction in a patient with severe primary pulmonary hypertension. Anesthesiology 1999;91(6):1943–5.

58. Fischer LG, Van Aken H, Bürkle H. Management of pulmonary hypertension: physiological and pharmacological considerations for anesthesiologists. Anesth Analg 2003;96(6):1603–6.

59. Biondi JW, Schulman DS, Soufer R, et al. The effect of incremental positive end-expiratory pressure on right ventricular hemodynamics and ejection fraction. Anesth Analg 1988;67(2):144–51.

60. Pritts CD, Pearl RG. Anesthesia for patients with pulmonary hypertension. Curr Opin Anaesthesiol 2010; 23(3):411–6.

61. Zamanian RT, Haddad F, Doyle RL WA. Management strategies for patients with pulmonary hypertension in the intensive care unit. Crit Care Med 2007;35:2037–50.

62. Sablotzki A, Starzmann W, Scheubel R. Selective pulmonary vasodilation with inhaled aerosolized milrinone in heart transplant candidates. Can J Anaesthesiol 2005;52:1076–82.

63. Michard F, Teboul J. Predicting fluid responsiveness in ICU patients: a critical analysis of the evidence. Chest 2002;121:2000–8.

Managing the Patient with Pulmonary Hypertension
Specialty Care Centers, Coordinated Care, and Patient Support

Murali M. Chakinala, MD[a],*, Maribeth Duncan, APRN[b],
Joel Wirth, MD[c,d]

KEYWORDS

- Pulmonary Hypertension Care Centers • Multidisciplinary care • Comanagement • Accreditation

KEY POINTS

- Pulmonary hypertension (PH) remains a challenging condition to detect, properly diagnose, and manage longitudinally in an era of ever-expanding therapies.
- The Pulmonary Hypertension Care Center program of the Pulmonary Hypertension Association was developed to address challenges in caring for patients with PH and improve the quality of care and long-term outcomes.
- Effective management of pulmonary arterial hypertension (PAH) requires close coordination between experienced practitioners from numerous disciplines at specialty referral centers and community-based practitioners.
- PAH patients' needs are best met by using the numerous health care resources that extend beyond the specialty care center.

INTRODUCTION

The field of pulmonary hypertension (PH) has evolved and expanded tremendously since the 1990s in conjunction with greater understanding of the condition, better appreciation of the epidemiology and, most important, the availability of numerous medical therapies specific for pulmonary arterial hypertension (PAH). In particular,

PAH (or group 1 PH of the 5th World Symposium on Pulmonary Hypertension) has been transformed from a fatal disease with a very limited life expectancy to a chronic, manageable condition with a lifespan that can last years to decades.[1] As PAH patients live longer, unique management issues have arisen and large cohorts of patients have been compiled at specialty centers throughout the country. This article builds

Disclosures: M.M. Chakinala is a member of the Pulmonary Hypertension Association's Scientific Leadership Council, a member of the Pulmonary Hypertension Care Center Oversight Committee, and is a paid reviewer of CME content for the Pulmonary Hypertension Association (under the supervision of the Washington University Office of Continuing Medical Education). M. Duncan has no relevant disclosures. J. Wirth is a member of the Pulmonary Hypertension Association's Scientific Leadership Council and a member of the Pulmonary Hypertension Care Center Review Committee.
a Division of Pulmonary and Critical Care Medicine, Washington University School of Medicine, 660 South Euclid Avenue, CB #8052, St Louis, MO 63110, USA; b Barnes-Jewish Hospital, One Barnes Jewish Hospital Plaza, St Louis, MO 63110, USA; c Department of Medicine, Tufts University School of Medicine, Boston, MA 02111, USA; d Division of Pulmonary and Critical Care Medicine, Maine Medical Center, Portland, ME 04012, USA
* Corresponding author.
E-mail address: chakinalam@wustl.edu

Cardiol Clin 34 (2016) 489–500
http://dx.doi.org/10.1016/j.ccl.2016.04.008
0733-8651/16/$ – see front matter © 2016 Elsevier Inc. All rights reserved.

on many of the medical and scientific concepts that are relevant to this issue, by discussing evolving health care delivery for PH using a model of specialty centers staffed by multidisciplinary teams who strive to co-manage patients with local community-based physicians.

CURRENT CHALLENGES IN THE MANAGEMENT OF PULMONARY HYPERTENSION
Centralized Versus Decentralized Care

Historically in the United States (and still in many parts of the world), the care of PAH patients followed a centralized model with prompt referral of newly diagnosed patients to expert centers for comprehensive evaluation, accurate diagnosis, and access to advanced therapies, such as intravenous prostacyclin by home-based continuous infusion and lung transplantation. With greater awareness of PAH and development of many simpler pharmacologic options, management of PAH has shifted from tertiary referral centers to a broader range of health care providers and facilities thus leading to decentralized care. Concomitantly, PAH-specific therapies have been applied to increasingly diverse patients within group 1 PH and sometimes to non–group 1 PH patients, often leading to predictably poor treatment responses or even potential harm while increasing health care expenditures.

According to the Rare Disease Act of 2002 and the National Organization for Rare Disorders, any condition that affects fewer than 200,000 individuals at any given time in the United States constitutes a rare disease.[2] Multiple national registries (conducted outside of the United States) assert a prevalence of 15 to 26 cases of PAH per million inhabitants, thus making PAH a rare disease in the United States and the developed world.[3–5] However, World Health Organization diagnostic groups 2 and 3 PH are very common conditions encountered in the context of underlying cardiac or pulmonary disorders, such as heart failure, valvular heart disease, chronic obstructive pulmonary disease, interstitial disease, and obstructive sleep apnea. In fact, PAH represents a very uncommon form of PH that can be diagnosed only after a comprehensive evaluation to exclude other types of PH, especially the more prevalent group 2 and group 3 varieties.[6]

Challenges in Evaluating Pulmonary Hypertension and Diagnostic Errors

The evaluation of PH is a multistep and laborious process.[7] Challenges to completing thorough and accurate evaluations in patients suspected of having PH include the inability to perform some of the most critical diagnostic studies (eg, ventilation–perfusion scans and right heart catheterizations) as well as a lack of sufficient experience to analyze certain diagnostic studies, especially echocardiograms and the hemodynamic data from invasive right heart catheterization, both of which require a thorough understanding of the pertinent pathophysiology and adherence to strict protocols of measurement (**Table 1**).

Recent publications have shed light on some emerging challenges relative to overdiagnosis errors. In A Multi-Center Study Of The Referral Of Pulmonary Hypertension Patients To Tertiary Pulmonary Hypertension Centers (RePHerral) Study, conducted at 3 large university-based tertiary care referral centers in the United States, 98 of 140 referred patients had been assigned a definitive diagnosis of PAH before referral, but 32 (33%) were ultimately determined to be misdiagnosed. Fifty-nine patients had not undergone a prereferral right heart catheterization. Forty-two patients were started on PAH-specific medications before referral, but contrary to published guidelines in more than one-half of the instances.[8] The PAH Quality Enhancement Research Initiative project revealed underuse of guideline-mandated studies for the evaluation of PH, especially the ventilation–perfusion scan and right heart catheterization, which can greatly impact the ultimate PH diagnosis and treatment approach.[9]

Challenges with the Management of Pulmonary Arterial Hypertension

Medical treatment options have truly revolutionized the care of PAH patients. Presently, there are 13 medications from 4 different classes of therapies—endothelin receptor antagonists, phosphodiesterase 5 inhibitors, soluble guanylate cyclase stimulators, and prostacyclin modulators—approved by the United States Federal Drug Administration. Although all medications have been proven efficacious, numerous factors distinguish the agents, including route of administration, ease of drug delivery, side effect profile, and cost, leading to variable use of medications. Indeed, the simplicity of oral agents makes them the most commonly used, even though more complex parenteral therapies are quite effective and considered the preferred treatment for the most compromised individuals.[10,11] Furthermore, combination regimens with drugs from more than one class are increasingly being used based on the findings of recent large-scale studies.[10–15]

Table 1
Challenges with the diagnostic evaluation of pulmonary hypertension

Diagnostic Study	Role in PH Management	Challenges to Proper Use	Potential Consequences
Ventilation-perfusion scan	Screening test for CTEPH	Unavailability at some facilities Supplanted by CT Angiography based on acute pulmonary embolism experience	Reliance on CT angiogram Underrecognition of chronic thromboembolic disease
Echocardiogram	Initial study for evaluation of dyspnea or right-sided heart failure Assessing prognosis and determining treatment Monitoring response to treatment	Poor visualization of the Tricuspid regurgitation jet and poor estimate of right atrial pressures Underappreciation of left ventricular diastolic dysfunction Difficulty assessing right ventricular dimensions and function Difficulty tracking right ventricular characteristics over time	Underrecognition of PH Misclassifying group 2 PH as group 1 PH Condition's severity may be misjudged and treatment choice impacted Fail to identify early worsening of condition
Functional class assessment	Global assessment of the condition's impact on an individual Assessing prognosis and determining treatment Monitoring response to treatment	Vague definitions of functional classes lead to inaccuracy Lack of standardized method for assessing lead to inadequate intergrader agreement	Misjudgment of PAH severity that may impact treatment Failure to capture early worsening of an individual's condition
6-Minute walk test	Assessment of exercise capacity Assessing prognosis and determining treatment Monitoring response to treatment	Not adhering to standardized protocol for study performance Not performing on consistent basis Confounding factors affecting test performance	Compromised accuracy and reliability of data Failure to capture early worsening of condition Diminished ability to assess condition and make treatment decision
Right heart catheterization	Confirm diagnosis of PAH Exclude left-sided cardiac conditions that lead to group 2 PH Assessing prognosis and determining treatment Monitoring response to treatment	Inability to perform procedure Not adhering to recommendations for accurate measurement of hemodynamics Relying on computer-generated pressure measurements in lieu of manual waveform interpretations Inaccuracy of measuring left-sided filling pressures (PAWP or LVEDP) Inability to perform acute vasodilator testing when IPAH suspected	Unable to make a definitive PAH diagnosis and possibly miscategorizing between groups 1 and 2 PH Not detecting acute vasoresponders who can be successfully treated with calcium channel blockers

Abbreviations: CT, computed tomography; CTEPH, chronic thromboembolic pulmonary hypertension; LVEDP, left ventricular end-diastolic pressure; PAH, pulmonary arterial hypertension; PAWP, pulmonary artery wedge pressure; PH, pulmonary hypertension.

Treatment algorithms borne out of complex evidence-based rubrics are widely available and recommend risk stratifying PAH patients to optimally tailor treatment regimens based on the severity of an individual's condition.[10,11,16] Despite the availability of evidence-based treatment recommendations, additional literature spotlights some shortcomings in the management of PAH patients. Evidence suggests that PAH patients followed outside of a referral center (compared with individuals already under the referral center's care) may be undertreated; oral therapies are used for longer periods before initiation of parenteral prostanoids, which may have contributed to a more compromised state. There was an increased need for urgent initiation of parenteral prostanoids and lesser survival rates observed in these patients, even after prostanoids were initiated.[17] This raises the question of whether reliance on oral therapies by nonexpert centers delayed the appropriate and timely use of parenteral prostanoids.

Once initiated on therapy, PAH patients require close monitoring to ensure achievement of appropriate treatment goals.[18,19] Patients also require surveillance for either inadequate treatment response or early identification of clinical progression, both of which presages unwanted clinical outcomes such as hospitalization, urgent initiation of advanced therapies, or possibly death.[20–22] Although the method of follow-up, namely the type of objective data, varies to some degree, published recommendations include many of the same studies used to diagnose PAH leading to the same inherent challenges described previously (see **Table 1**).[19]

Although many of these reports have shortcomings in terms of their small scale, retrospective design, or missing data, they consistently underscore the perceptions of late recognition of PH, inaccurate diagnosis of PAH, untimely referral to expert centers, and underuse of advanced therapies. Given these evolving shortcomings and the growing challenges of managing PAH patients in the long-term, there has been a pressing need to refocus care for this rare and complex disorder. In essence, reemphasis on the specialty center and a shift towards more centralized care has been an aim for many vested stakeholders in the PH community, following the lead of other rare disease groups such as cystic fibrosis, hemophilia, and Marfan syndrome, among many others.[23]

SPECIALTY CARE CENTERS
The Evidence for Team-based Care in Chronic Disease Management

Multidisciplinary team-based patient care has been noted widely to be an important strategy to improve health care quality.[24,25] The Institute of Medicine has noted, "To close the gaps between best practice and usual care … will require the collective expertise of a vast array of doctors, nurses, pharmacists, allied health professionals, social workers, and vested laypersons."[26] Team-based health care has been defined as "the provision of health services to individuals, families, and/or their communities by at least two healthcare providers who work collaboratively with patients and their caregivers – to the extent preferred by each patient – to accomplish shared goals within and across settings to achieve coordinated, high-quality care."[27] It has been shown that multidisciplinary health care teams are clinically effective and can improve the quality of clinical care delivered in a spectrum of acute and chronic care settings.[28] Key factors for successful team-based care include clinical and administrative systems, division of labor, team member training, effective communication, incorporating measurable outcomes, and leadership.[29] Wagner and colleagues[28] noted that effective team care exploits multiple strategies including population-based care, treatment planning, evidence-based clinical management, self-management support, and effective use of consultation. Coordinators (often defined as nurse case managers) have been used generally for patient self-management education, enhancing communication, and implementing behavioral therapies. A recent metaanalysis highlighted the significant contribution of clinical pharmacist–physician collaboration in a wide spectrum of chronic diseases. Specifically, improvements have been demonstrated in medication safety as well as clinical outcomes and patient centered outcomes (medication adherence, patient knowledge and quality of life–general health scores).[30]

Designing the Pulmonary Hypertension Care Center Program: Key Goals and Features

A principal goal of the Pulmonary Hypertension Association (PHA) Pulmonary Hypertension Care Center (PHCC) program is to function as a national quality improvement project: to better define and promote PAH standards of care in an effort to improve patient outcomes. Its mission statement states, "The purpose of the Pulmonary Hypertension Care Centers initiative is to establish a program of accredited centers with expertise in PH that aspires to improve overall quality of care and ultimately improve outcomes of patients with PH, particularly PAH, a rare and life-threatening disease."[31] The program has been structured to align professionals, patients, and caregivers to enhance awareness of PH disease, increase access to expert care, promote adherence to published diagnosis and management guidelines, support collaboration among clinical programs to optimize PAH clinical management and research, and to grow the PH community.

Improving Access to Expert Pulmonary Hypertension Care and Supporting Collaboration Among Clinical Programs

The PHCC Program was designed to encompass both Centers of Comprehensive Care (CCC) and Regional Clinical Programs. These designations are based on the resources available and therapies offered by each program (**Table 2**). The rationale behind creating a multitiered program is to optimize access to expert care for PH patients and caregivers. Indeed, patients with unexplained PH, PAH patients not meeting current multifaceted treatment goals, or patients with severe PH in the setting of chronic heart or lung disease, are worthy candidates for early referral to a PHCC. Careful consideration was given to balancing the goal of reasonable geographic access for patients with the goal of accrediting centers with adequate PH expertise and resources. Currently, few data exist to define the optimal program size, resources, and experience needed to provide safe and effective care to patients with PH. The PHCC Program hopes to help define these program attributes in the future.

Collaboration between the Regional Clinical Programs and CCCs for both clinical care and research is highly encouraged and integral to the PHCC program. In addition to adult programs (both CCC and Regional Clinical Program), pediatric CCC programs have defined specific attributes appropriate to their PH patient population.

Promoting Adherence to Published Diagnosis and Management Guidelines, Optimizing the Clinical Management of Pulmonary Arterial Hypertension, and Research

The PHCC Program seeks to promote a multidisciplinary team approach to PH care. The important role of appropriately experienced physician and allied health personnel to coordinate the care of this complex patient population is recognized and integral to the program structure. Each PHCC must have appropriate resources and institutional support, education and training of core staff, ancillary services, protocols for the safe management of PAH patients, and adequate inpatient and outpatient facilities. The PHCC organization was designed to promote principles of population-based care, evidence-based PH diagnosis and management, and to support patient self-management through education and involvement in patient support groups. Another key feature of the program is use of effective consultation relative to transplantation, pulmonary thromboendarterectomy surgery, and palliative care.

By better understanding and studying regional differences in care, the program seeks to promote best practices and reduce unwanted variations in PH care. As a key tool to support quality improvement, the PHA Registry was launched in August 2015. The expressed goals of the PHA Registry are to collect data from each PHCC to assess outcomes with an aim of improving both quality of life and survival for patients with PAH and chronic thromboembolic pulmonary hypertension. As the registry matures and develops nationally, it holds great promise in defining, refining, and promoting safe and effective PH care.

The capacity to participate in PH-related clinical research is also a core feature of each PHA comprehensive care center to help meet the goals of improving the quality of patients' lives and working towards a cure for PH (particularly PAH). Each PHCC comprehensive care center has sufficient research infrastructure and a demonstrated history of clinical research and academic productivity. The PHCC Regional Clinical Programs help to promote clinical research through program collaboration and appropriate subject identification.

Table 2
Categories of Pulmonary Hypertension Care Centers

	Center for Comprehensive Care (CCC)	Regional Clinical Program (RCP)
Center director	***	**
Center coordinator	***	**
Program staff and support services	***	*
Facilities	***	*
Patient-oriented research	**	—

Asterisks indicate number and breadth of criteria in a category.

Promoting Pulmonary Hypertension Disease Awareness and Growing the Pulmonary Hypertension Community

Involvement in community outreach and education are also core elements of the PHCC program. Participation in local, regional, national, and international educational events relative to PH is strongly encouraged. Community outreach, broadly defined, is a key focus for each PHCC, and can take many forms. Ongoing patient and caregiver educational efforts help support the goal of effective patient self-management.

The PHCC program seeks to be inclusionary to help grow the PH community nationwide. Through development and support of both larger and smaller programs as well as fostering active program collaboration, the program seeks to attract all with the shared goals and objectives of improving the lives of patients with PH.

The Pulmonary Hypertension Care Center Accreditation Process

The initial PHCC accreditation criteria have focused on the evaluation of PH patients, diagnosis of PAH, and appropriate use of therapies for group I (PAH) and group IV (chronic thromboembolic pulmonary hypertension) patients (**Boxes 1** and **2**) highlight some of the principal elements assessed at each prospective site and also reflect the structure and functions of an active PHCC.[32]

The rationale leading to the development of the PHCC accreditation program and its implementation have recently been reviewed.[23,33] The PHA accreditation program assesses each facility's resources, including required ancillary services, education and training of core staff, protocols for the safe management of PAH patients, and inpatient and outpatient facilities.

The process for accreditation of PHCC programs includes multiple evaluation elements. Beyond the structural and contextual elements described, all PHA-accredited programs are evaluated regarding their ability to provide appropriate and effective care to PH patients. Applicants are required to complete an online application, obtain letters of support from ancillary program services, assemble supporting documents, and help to coordinate a 1-day site visit. The PHCC Review Committee members perform site visits during which PH program faculty, staff, and patients are interviewed. Topics for review include clinical and administrative support systems, division of labor, team member training, effectiveness of communication, and leadership.

In addition, a focused chart review aimed at evaluating PH diagnosis and management is performed with the assistance of the program leadership. Programs are assessed regarding compliance with broadly accepted diagnostic and management guidelines with appropriate delivery of PAH and chronic thromboembolic pulmonary hypertension specific therapies.

Participation by the site personnel in community outreach and education are also assessed. Capacity to participate in clinical research is reviewed at prospective CCC programs. Programs need to substantially satisfy the established PHCC criteria for successful accreditation.[34] The PHCC attempts to be flexible in evaluating how individual programs provide individualized care within their local environments. As of December 2015, more than 30 CCC programs have been accredited in the United States.

BEYOND THE SPECIALTY CARE CENTER
Long-term Comanagement of the Patient with Pulmonary Arterial Hypertension

Long-term management of PAH patients revolves around several key issues. First and foremost, patients require close surveillance of right ventricular function to facilitate the early detection of progressive right-sided heart failure, which is key to survival in PAH and leads to important consequences, including hospitalization, need for advanced medical therapies, or referral for lung transplantation. Additionally, management should focus on optimizing pulmonary vasomodulators, including the selection of medications and appropriate dosing, while minimizing side effects and risk of complications (eg, prostanoid-related side effects or catheter-related bloodstream infection). The long-term management of PAH also requires attention to comorbid conditions that can impact an individual's condition and potentially limit the benefits of PAH therapies; some of these comorbid conditions are related directly to the underlying cause of PAH such as in systemic sclerosis, portal hypertension associated with cirrhosis, or congenital heart disease, and may have great relevance (**Box 3**, **Table 3**). Finally, general medical follow-up for common medical ailments and customary cancer screening that is age and gender appropriate, when life expectancy is at least 5 years, is becoming increasingly important because patients are living years, if not decades, after PAH is diagnosed.

Clearly, comprehensive management of the PAH patient is challenging and difficult for a

Box 1
Center for comprehensive care

Center director
- Board certified in pulmonary medicine, critical care, or cardiology
- 2 years of experience treating PAH after training
- At least 50% of director's effort dedicated to PH center
- 30 hours of CME related to PH over past 3 years
- Involved in PH-related education

Center coordinator
- Licensed allied health care professional (RN, NP, PA, RRT, or pharmacist)
- Proficiency with all PAH therapies
- Involved in PH-related education
- 12 hours of CME/CEU related to PH over past 3 years

Program staff and support services
- Center managing a minimum of 75 patients with PAH or CTEPH
- Experience administering all PAH therapies
- Adequate experience with parenteral prostanoid infusions
- Adheres to available diagnosis and treatment consensus guidelines
- Outpatient nursing support commensurate with the center's patient volume
- Availability of relevant consultants

Facilities
- PH team directly involved with care of inpatients
- Inpatient wards and ICUs trained to manage PAH patients
- Cardiac catheterization laboratory capable of acute vasodilator testing
- Echocardiography laboratory with experience imaging PH and the right ventricle
- Pulmonary function laboratory capable of performing exercise testing
- Pharmacy with immediate access to parenteral prostacyclin analogues
- Radiology department with expertise in imaging PH
- Institutional support for the center

Research
- Program participated in patient-oriented clinical research
- Knowledgeable research staff
- Investigational drug service
- Center staff has PH-related publication within the last 5 years

Abbreviations: CEU, continuing education unit; CME, continuing medical education; CTEPH, chronic thromboembolic pulmonary hypertension; ICU, intensive care unit; NP, nurse practitioner; PA, physician assistant; PAH, pulmonary arterial hypertension; PH, pulmonary hypertension; RN, registered nurse; RRT, registered respiratory therapist.
For a complete listing of criteria, see reference.[32]

specialty center to solely manage, especially because many patients do not live in close proximity to a specialty center. The ideal framework for coping with these complex and interrelated issues is a collaborative relationship between the specialty center and local health care practitioners (HCPs), both groups taking an active and complementary role in management. Although specific responsibilities between the different parties can vary based on their unique practice environments and geography, a general framework is suggested in **Fig. 1**.

Box 2
Regional Clinical Programs

Center director
- Board certified in pulmonary medicine, critical care, or cardiology
- 2 years of experience treating PAH after training
- 20 hours of CME related to PH over past 3 years
- Involved in PH-related education

Center coordinator
- Licensed allied health care professional (RN, NP, PA, RRT, or pharmacist)
- Proficiency with non-parenteral PAH therapies
- Involved in PH-related education
- 12 hours of CME/CEU related to PH over past 3 years

Program staff and support services
- Center managing a minimum of 25 patients with PAH or CTEPH
- Experience administering all nonparenteral PAH therapies
- Adheres to available diagnosis and treatment consensus guidelines
- Outpatient nursing support commensurate with the center's patient volume
- Availability of relevant consultants
- Collaborates and comanages patients with regional CCC

Facilities
- PH team directly involved with care of inpatients
- ICU facilities within affiliated hospital
- Cardiac catheterization laboratory capable of acute vasodilator testing
- Echocardiography laboratory with experience imaging PH and the right ventricle
- Radiology department with expertise in imaging PH
- Pulmonary function laboratory capable of performing exercise testing

Abbreviations: CCC, Center for comprehensive care; CEU, continuing education unit; CME, continuing medical education; CTEPH, chronic thromboembolic pulmonary hypertension; ICU, intensive care unit; NP, nurse practitioner; PA, physician assistant; PAH, pulmonary arterial hypertension; PH, pulmonary hypertension; RN, registered nurse; RRT, registered respiratory therapist.

External Organizations

Outside of the specialty care center and community-based practitioners, several external groups have distinct roles in the long-term management of PAH patients. These various entities provide invaluable and unique services that supplement the efforts of the PH team, and in some cases, directly implement treatment plans.

PAH has witnessed tremendous growth in the number of medical therapies over the past decade. The arsenal of therapeutic options has positively impacted survival and prognosis for patients with PAH. Because of drug cost, complexity, and need for risk mitigation, much

of the available therapies are dispensed through specialty pharmacies, which focus on high-cost, high-touch medications for patients with complex disease states. Typically, specialty pharmacies provide patients necessary training, education, and support necessary to manage complicated therapies, and assist practitioners with risk mitigation strategies. Their nurses train patients, caregivers, and HCPs in the management and administration of complex PH-specific therapies, in particular parenteral therapies. Pharmacists also assist with patient education and counseling regarding therapies. Specialty pharmacies insurance and reimbursement specialists communicate directly with

Box 3
Comorbid conditions associated with underlying cause of pulmonary arterial hypertension

Systemic sclerosis
- Iron-deficiency anemia
- Gastroesophageal reflux
- Gastrointestinal dysmotility
- Raynaud's/digital ulcers
- Interstitial lung disease

Portal hypertension/cirrhosis
- Gastrointestinal bleeding
- Thrombocytopenia
- Ascites
- Encephalopathy

Congenital heart disease
- Complex anatomic defects
- Arrhythmia
- Hyperuricemia
- Hyperviscosity
- Hemoptysis
- Thrombocytopenia

patients and HCP offices to troubleshoot issues in the referral process. According to the American Pharmacists Association, enlisting a specialty-trained pharmacist as part of the

Table 3
Medical conditions impacting patients with pulmonary arterial hypertension

Condition	Recommendation
Chronic kidney disease	Avoiding nephrotoxins Monitoring renal function Optimizing diuretic use
Iron-deficiency anemia	Monitoring hemoglobin Iron supplementation, as needed Caution with medications that promote bleeding
Arrhythmias	Prompt recognition Consider early restoration of sinus rhythm
Physical deconditioning	Formal exercise training Encourage regular activity
Depression	Screen for symptoms Counseling and psychotherapy Pharmacotherapy

collaborative care team enhances patient satisfaction, reduces complications of drug treatment, reduces use of unnecessary medications, improves laboratory monitoring, and helps to control costs.[35]

Durable medical equipment companies are also widely used in the PH population as with any chronic medical condition. Their primary role is to provide equipment to aid in better quality of living, including long-term oxygen delivery systems, positive pressure ventilation devices, and ambulatory assistance devices, hospital beds.

Nonprofit organizations represent another crucial external group that provides extensive assistance to PAH patients and aids the efforts of HCPs. Two such groups are the PHA and Caring Voice Coalition. PHA is the result of a grassroots effort to create a national network for patients. PHA has grown to a community of well over 10,000 PH patients, caregivers, family members, and medical professionals. Despite its growth to as many as 50 PH Associations worldwide, PHA has stayed true to its original mission of support, education, advocacy, and awareness (**Box 4**). The education focus has been met through a variety of live programs, printed materials including the *Pulmonary Hypertension – A Patients Survival Guide*, and online instruments. Meanwhile, networking opportunities exist for patients through dozens of local support groups across the country and for health care professionals via PH Clinicians and Researchers Network and the PH Professional Network. Caring Voice Coalition is another nonprofit organization that offers outreach services including financial, emotional, and educational support. Their Insurance Education and Counseling program provides 4 basic services: reviewing and explaining benefits, mediating problems and complaints, exploring new or improved coverage, and helping with Social Security Disability applications.

Lastly, pharmaceutical-sponsored patient assistance programs provide eligible patients with access to medications at reduced or deferred cost. PH drug manufacturers offer programs with varying levels of assistance, including copay assistance, coupon programs, and even total financial coverage to ensure drug availability in hardship cases; many of the pharmaceutical companies also donate to the Caring Voice Coalition, which in turn awards patients need-based grants for meeting their health care costs. In addition, many of the pharmaceutical companies provide educational programs geared toward the lay public, focusing on the disease state and PAH treatments.

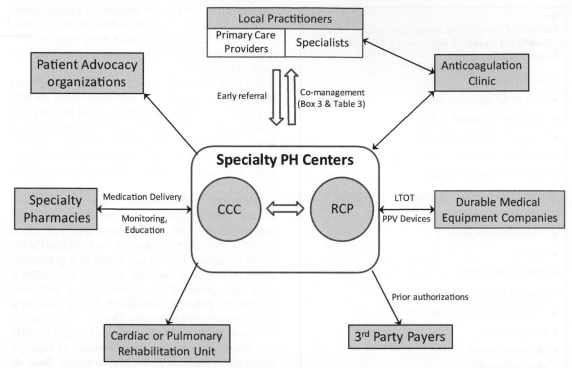

Fig. 1. A proposed scheme for coordinating care of patients with pulmonary hypertension (PH) between specialty care centers, community-based practitioners, and third-party organizations with a vested interest in the care of patients with pulmonary arterial hypertension (PAH). The exact relationship in individual cases will depend on the scope services performed by community-based practitioners, proximity to the specialty care PH center, patient's preferences, and restrictions from third-party payers. CCC, comprehensive care center; LTOT, long-term oxygen therapy; PPV, positive pressure ventilation; RCP, regional clinical program.

Box 4
Pulmonary Hypertension Association services

For patients
- Support groups
- PHA online classroom
- Biennial international conference
- Regional 'on the road' conferences
- Legislation advocacy
- Phone and online support
- *Pulmonary Hypertension – A Patients Survival Guide*

For health care practitioners
- Medical education programs
- Continuing medical education
- Professional networks
- Pulmonary Hypertension Association online university
- *Advances in Pulmonary Hypertension*

SUMMARY

Despite remarkable advances in the last 20 years, PH remains a very complex and lethal condition that is often misunderstood and misdiagnosed. The availability of numerous therapies for PAH challenges HCPs to use treatments appropriately, toward improving long-term outcomes. As PAH patients live longer, their care becomes even more complex and demanding owing to the potential for long-term comorbidities and general medical problems. Despite these challenges, PAH care in the United States has become more decentralized and shortcomings in its diagnosis and management have emerged. The PHA-sponsored PHCC program, which was developed to recognize centers providing multidisciplinary and comprehensive care, is refocusing the spotlight on specialty care centers, which have been successful in other rare diseases. As a quality improvement initiative, the PHCC program also hopes to raise the standard of care for PAH patients across the country. Optimizing long-term care of PAH patients will require well-coordinated comanagement between specialty care centers, community-based practitioners, ancillary services and programs, patients, and care givers.

REFERENCES

1. Simonneau G, Gatzoulis MA, Adatia I, et al. Updated clinical classification of pulmonary hypertension. J Am Coll Cardiol 2013;62(Suppl 25):D34–41.
2. Rare Diseases Act of 2002. In: NOoR, editor. Disorders; 2002. p. 1988–1991.
3. Humbert M, Sitbon O, Chaouat A, et al. Pulmonary arterial hypertension in France: results from a national registry. Am J Respir Crit Care Med 2006; 173(9):1023–30.
4. Escribano-Subias P, Blanco I, Lopez-Meseguer M, et al. Survival in pulmonary hypertension in Spain: insights from the Spanish registry. Eur Respir J 2012;40(3):596–603.
5. Peacock AJ, Murphy NF, McMurray JJ, et al. An epidemiological study of pulmonary arterial hypertension. Eur Respir J 2007;30(1):104–9.
6. Strange G, Playford D, Stewart S, et al. Pulmonary hypertension: prevalence and mortality in the Armadale echocardiography cohort. Heart 2012;98(24): 1805–11.
7. Hoeper MM, Bogaard HJ, Condliffe R, et al. Definitions and diagnosis of pulmonary hypertension. J Am Coll Cardiol 2013;62(Suppl 25):D42–50.
8. Deano RC, Glassner-Kolmin C, Rubenfire M, et al. Referral of patients with pulmonary hypertension diagnoses to tertiary pulmonary hypertension centers: the multicenter RePHerral study. JAMA Intern Med 2013;173(10):887–93.
9. McLaughlin VV, Langer A, Tan M, et al. Contemporary trends in the diagnosis and management of pulmonary arterial hypertension: an initiative to close the care gap. Chest 2013;143(2):324–32.
10. Galie N, Corris PA, Frost A, et al. Updated treatment algorithm of pulmonary arterial hypertension. J Am Coll Cardiol 2013;62(Suppl 25):D60–72.
11. Galie N, Humbert M, Vachiery JL, et al. 2015 ESC/ERS Guidelines for the diagnosis and treatment of pulmonary hypertension: The Joint Task Force for the Diagnosis and Treatment of Pulmonary Hypertension of the European Society of Cardiology (ESC) and the European Respiratory Society (ERS)Endorsed by: Association for European Paediatric and Congenital Cardiology (AEPC), International Society for Heart and Lung Transplantation (ISHLT). Eur Heart J 2015;37(1): 67–119.
12. Pulido T, Adzerikho I, Channick RN, et al. Macitentan and morbidity and mortality in pulmonary arterial hypertension. N Engl J Med 2013;369(9):809–18.
13. Galie N, Barbera JA, Frost AE, et al. Initial use of ambrisentan plus tadalafil in pulmonary arterial hypertension. N Engl J Med 2015;373(9):834–44.
14. McLaughlin VV, Benza RL, Rubin LJ, et al. Addition of inhaled treprostinil to oral therapy for pulmonary arterial hypertension: a randomized controlled clinical trial. J Am Coll Cardiol 2010; 55(18):1915–22.
15. Ghofrani HA, Galie N, Grimminger F, et al. Riociguat for the treatment of pulmonary arterial hypertension. N Engl J Med 2013;369(4):330–40.
16. Taichman DB, Ornelas J, Chung L, et al. Pharmacologic therapy for pulmonary arterial hypertension in adults: CHEST guideline and expert panel report. Chest 2014;146(2):449–75.
17. Badagliacca R, Pezzuto B, Poscia R, et al. Prognostic factors in severe pulmonary hypertension patients who need parenteral prostanoid therapy: the impact of late referral. J Heart Lung Transplant 2012;31(4):364–72.
18. McLaughlin VV, Gaine SP, Howard LS, et al. Treatment goals of pulmonary hypertension. J Am Coll Cardiol 2013;62(Suppl 25):D73–81.
19. McLaughlin VV, Archer SL, Badesch DB, et al. ACCF/AHA 2009 expert consensus document on pulmonary hypertension: a report of the American College of Cardiology Foundation Task Force on Expert Consensus Documents and the American Heart Association: developed in collaboration with the American College of Chest Physicians, American Thoracic Society, Inc., and the Pulmonary Hypertension Association. Circulation 2009;119(16): 2250–94.
20. Burger CD, Long PK, Shah MR, et al. Characterization of first-time hospitalizations in patients with newly diagnosed pulmonary arterial hypertension in the REVEAL registry. Chest 2014;146(5): 1263–73.
21. Farber HW, Miller DP, McGoon MD, et al. Predicting outcomes in pulmonary arterial hypertension based on the 6-minute walk distance. J Heart Lung Transplant 2015;34(3):362–8.
22. Farber HW, Miller DP, Poms AD, et al. Five-year outcomes of patients enrolled in the REVEAL registry. Chest 2015;148(4):1043–54.
23. Chakinala MM, McGoon M. Pulmonary hypertension care centers: it's time has come. Adv Pulm Hypertens 2014;12(4):175–8.
24. Yarnall KS, Ostbye T, Krause KM, et al. Family physicians as team leaders: "time" to share the care. Prev Chronic Dis 2009;6(2):A59.
25. Mitchell P, Wynia M, Golden R, et al. Core principles and values of team-based health care. Washington, DC: Institute of Medicine; 2012.
26. Adams K, Corrigan J. Priority areas for national action. Washington, DC: The National Academy Press; 2003.

27. Naylor MD, Coburn KD, Kurtzman ET, et al. Inter-professional team-based primary care for chronically ill adults: State of the science. ABIM Foundation Meeting To Advance Team-Based Care for the Chronically Ill in Ambulatory Settings. Philadelphia (PA), March 24-25, 2010.

28. Wagner EH, Austin BT, Davis C, et al. Improving chronic illness care: translating evidence into action. Health Aff 2001;20(6):64–78.

29. Grumbach K, Bodenheimer T. Can health care teams improve primary care practice? JAMA 2004; 291(10):1246–51.

30. Chisholm-Burns MA, Kim Lee J, Spivey CA, et al. US pharmacists' effect as team members on patient care: systematic review and meta-analyses. Med Care 2010;48(10):923–33.

31. Pulmonary Hypertension Association (PHA). Medical professionals. Available at: www.phassociation.org/PHCareCenters/MedicalProfessionals. Accessed May 16, 2016.

32. Pulmonary Hypertension Association (PHA). Accreditation criteria. Available at: www.phassociation.org/PHCareCenters/MedicalProfessionals/CenterCriteria. Accessed May 16, 2016.

33. Wirth JA, Poms AD. Implementation of the PHA pulmonary hypertension care centers accreditation program. Adv Pulm Hypertens 2014;13(1):40–1.

34. Berman-Rosenzweig E. Pulmonary hypertension care centers: role of the Review Committee. Adv Pulm Hypertens 2014;13(2):94–5.

35. American Pharmacists Association. Homepage on the Internet. Available at: www.pharmacist.com. Accessed May 16, 2016.

Index

Note: Page numbers of article titles are in **boldface** type.

Cardiol Clin 34 (2016) 501–505
http://dx.doi.org/10.1016/S0733-8651(16)30051-0
0733-8651/16/$ – see front matter

Moving?

Make sure your subscription moves with you!

To notify us of your new address, find your **Clinics Account Number** (located on your mailing label above your name), and contact customer service at:

Email: journalscustomerservice-usa@elsevier.com

800-654-2452 (subscribers in the U.S. & Canada)
314-447-8871 (subscribers outside of the U.S. & Canada)

Fax number: 314-447-8029

Elsevier Health Sciences Division
Subscription Customer Service
3251 Riverport Lane
Maryland Heights, MO 63043

*To ensure uninterrupted delivery of your subscription, please notify us at least 4 weeks in advance of move.

ELSEVIER

Printed and bound by CPI Group (UK) Ltd, Croydon, CR0 4YY

03/10/2024

01040299-0002